UNDERSTANDING
Parkinson's Disease

— *A Self-Help Guide* —

SECOND EDITION

David L. Cram, M.D.

Steven H. Schechter, M.D.

Xiao-Ke Gao, M.D.

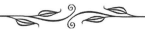

Addicus Books
Omaha, Nebraska

An Addicus Nonfiction Book

ISBN: 978-1-886039-00-1
Second Edition

Cover design by Michael Silverander
Illustrations by Jack Kusler
Typography by Linda Dageforde

This book is not intended to serve as a substitute for a physician, nor do the authors intend to give medical advice contrary to that of an attending physician.

Library of Congress Cataloging-in-Publication Data
Cram, David L. (David Lee), 1934-
    Understanding Parkinson's disease : a self-help guide /
    David L. Cram, Xiao-Ke Gao, Steven Schechter. — 2nd ed.
        p. cm.
    "An Addicus nonfiction book."
    Includes index.
    ISBN 978-1-886039-00-1 (alk. paper)
    1. Parkinson's disease—Popular works. I. Gao, Xiao Ke,
1953- II.
    Schechter, Steven, 1961- III. Title.
    RC382.C92 2009
    616.8'33—dc22   2009019976

Addicus Books, Inc.
www.AddicusBooks.com

10 9 8 7 6 5 4 3 2 1

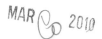 MAR 2010

To our daughter, Zoe Elizabeth,
who has brought us such love and joy.
—*Steven H. Schechter, M.D.*

To my mother, Yinming Huang
—*Xiao-Ke Gao, M.D.*

Contents

Introduction vii

1 A Self-Help Approach to Parkinson's Disease 1

2 What Is Parkinson's Disease? 4

3 The Emotional Side of Parkinson's Disease 18

4 Your Doctor as Partner 37

5 Drug Treatment for Parkinson's Disease 47

6 Surgery as Treatment for Parkinson's Disease . . . 64

7 The Importance of Exercise 71

8 Day-to-Day Coping 82

9 Caring for Caregivers 109

In Conclusion 123

Resources 124

Glossary 128

Index 138

About the Authors 145

Introduction

For those with a chronic, disabling neurological disorder such as Parkinson's disease, it is often hard to see a bright side to the adversity. Anger, self-pity, and fear may cloud your perceptions. You may feel so frightened that you give up. At times you might feel like a helpless victim, relying on others to perform even the most mundane tasks.

There is hope. Strides are being made to treat Parkinson's disease—thanks to new medications, surgical procedures, an active research community, health services, and support networks. One day, we may even have a cure.

The outlook for PD patients is considerably brighter today than it was even ten years ago. New medications are being developed. Services are available to make your life and the responsibilities of your caregivers easier. This book will help you understand Parkinson's disease, its various treatments, effective self-help strategies to feel better and remain physically active, and the many reasons for maintaining a cheerful outlook.

The world is full of suffering.
It's also full of overcoming it.

—Helen Keller
1880-1968

1

A Self-Help Approach to Parkinson's Disease

If you or someone you love has been diagnosed with Parkinson's disease (PD), it is easy to feel overwhelmed or believe there is nothing you can do. After all, PD is a chronic, progressive disease for which there is presently no cure. But, there *is* plenty you can do to improve your life or that of someone you love.

Self-help strategies can help improve the quality of life for those with PD. Self-help strategies can't cure the disease, but they can slow its progress and reduce the severity of symptoms. In addition, many new drugs can slow the progression and eliminate many aggravating symptoms. The self-help techniques offered here can help you maintain your independence for as long as possible. Perhaps most important, they can foster a sense of well-being and serenity in your life.

What Is Self-Help?

Self-help is a positive approach to your condition that says, "I have power. I have responsibility. I can make a difference in my disease." There are four important elements of self-help:

1. Attitude
2. Knowledge
3. Partnership with your doctors
4. Taking action

Attitude

Studies have repeatedly demonstrated that attitude can significantly affect a person's health. For example, research has found that people who are chronically hostile are more likely to suffer heart attacks. Our minds and bodies *are* connected. Although eating right, exercising, reducing stress, and getting enough rest are all important, your attitude is perhaps the most essential element of self-help.

We do not yet know how attitude affects the physical aspects of PD. For instance, we do not know whether an upbeat attitude only lessens symptoms or actually slows the progression of the disease. However, we do know that a positive attitude can improve the quality of your life. It *can* make you feel better. It can also enable you to take the self-help steps you need to keep feeling as good as you can for as long as you can.

Knowledge

Another essential tool of self-help is knowledge. It is important that you and your loved ones learn all you can about PD—what it is, what causes it, its symptoms, and treatment options. Stay abreast of the latest developments in research and treatment. Equipping yourselves with knowledge will reduce your fears and enable you to make the best-informed medical choices.

Partnership with Your Doctors

Self-help does not mean doing everything by and for yourself. Because you have a serious, progressive disease, your doctors must play a major role in your care. The old model of health care presumed that the doctor had all the power and made all the decisions concerning your medical treatment. By contrast, the self-help model acknowledges that you are an active partner with your doctors in your health care. Self-help comes with responsibilities. For instance, your doctors must select the right medicine in the correct dosage for your symptoms. Your job is to take the right amount of medication on time, keep track of your symptoms and side effects, let the doctors know how the medication is working, and report any problems you may be having with the treatment regimen.

Taking Action

Taking action means doing the things that make you feel better, slow the disability, and keep you independent for as long as possible. You can use specific self-help strategies to improve your diet, take your medications on time in the right amounts, reduce stress in your life, and get adequate rest. We will discuss each of these strategies further in the coming chapters.

By adopting a positive and upbeat attitude, equipping yourself with knowledge, partnering with your doctors, and taking action, you will give yourself the best possible chance at living better with PD.

2

What Is Parkinson's Disease?

Parkinson's disease is a progressive brain disorder. Doctors often call it a disorder of the *motor system*, which is the nerve system that controls body movement. Parkinson's disease (PD) occurs when brain cells, or *neurons*, decline and cause a deficiency of the brain chemical *dopamine*. This chemical (one of the brain's *neurotransmitters*) affects the part of the brain associated with muscle control, attention, learning, and the brain's pleasure and reward system. Low dopamine levels bring about the symptoms of PD.

Major Symptoms

Symptoms vary from person to person. For example, a certain symptom may develop early in one patient but develop much later (or never) in another patient. Symptoms may come on quickly or very gradually. In fact, sometimes the symptoms can be subtle and a person won't notice them for months or longer. Symptoms may affect one or both sides of the body. Often, a symptom will start on one side of the body and become more pronounced on that side.

Tremor

Trembling can affect the hands, arms, legs, jaw, and face. The classic PD tremor is a rhythmic back-and-forth movement of the thumb and forefinger, sometimes described as "pill rolling" because the tremor resembles the action of rolling a pill between the forefinger and thumb. The tremor usually begins in the hand but may also begin in the foot or jaw. About 75 percent of people with PD develop tremor; in the early stages of the disease, the tremor affects only one side of the body. The remaining 25 percent of PD patients never develop significant tremor.

Stiffness or Rigidity

For the body to move smoothly, opposing sets of muscles must alternately relax and contract. In a person with PD, muscles of the limbs and trunk may remain constantly tense and contracted. This may cause aching, stiffness, weakness, and jerky movements.

Slowness of Movement

Called *bradykinesia*, slowness of movement is an unpredictable and frustrating symptom of PD. One moment, you move easily. The next, you need help. Simple tasks, such as dressing, that were once performed easily may become difficult and time consuming.

Impaired Balance and Coordination

This symptom may prevent someone with PD from performing certain motor functions, making the individual fall easily or have a stooped posture. These symptoms tend to worsen over time. Eventually, the person with PD may experience difficulty walking, talking, or completing otherwise simple tasks.

Midbrain View of the Substantia Nigra

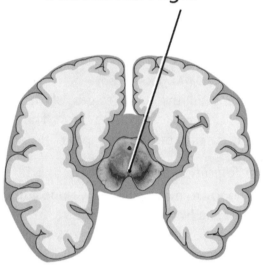

Normal Substantia Nigra

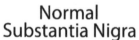

Diminished Substantia Nigra

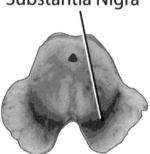

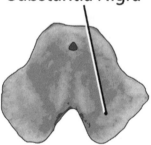

The top illustration shows the substantia nigra, a part of the brain involved in the release of neurons called dopamine, which help control muscle movement. The lower-left illustration is a close-up of a normal substantia nigra. The illustration on the lower right shows a diminished substantia nigra, found with Parkinson's disease.

Other Possible Symptoms

Depression and Emotional Changes

It is common, especially early in the disease, for people with PD to develop depression. Drugs used to treat PD symptoms sometimes worsen depression. However, some antidepressant drugs may safely and effectively be taken alongside these drugs.

Insecurity and fear are often secondary symptoms of PD. Some people with PD may feel that they can't cope with new situations and will therefore refuse to travel or socialize.

Pain

It's believed that nearly half of all PD patients experience some form of pain related to their PD. However, the discussion of pain as a symptom is often overlooked; patients often think the pain is caused by other factors. The pain commonly associated with PD is muscle pain, which can be caused by poor posture, rigidity, and lack of physical activity; backache is an example of pain that may occur as a result of these factors.

Pain may also be caused by *dystonia*, which is a neurological muscle disorder that causes uncontrollable muscle spasms resulting in abnormal movements and postures. A potentially painful condition, it can affect arms, legs, trunk, neck, face, tongue, jaw, or vocal cords. PD medications and physical activity help relieve dystonia.

Memory Loss/Slow Thinking

Although reasoning remains clear, it may be harder for someone with PD to remember or come up with solutions to problems as quickly as in the past.

Problems Swallowing/Chewing

In the later stages of PD, the throat muscles are less efficient, making it difficult to swallow or chew. Fortunately, medications can usually solve these difficulties.

Freezing

Freezing is a temporary inability to move that is common in people with advanced stages of PD. It is as if someone hit an "off" switch and movement stops. A person may have trouble getting up from a chair or it may seem as if a foot has become stuck to the floor. Freezing usually lasts only a few seconds or minutes, but because it is unpredictable, it can contribute to falls.

Changes in Speech

People with PD may experience changes in speech: rapid speech, slurred or repeated words, hesitation in speaking, or speaking too softly or in a monotone. Speech therapy can often help a person with PD cope with these problems.

Impaired Sense of Smell

A reduced sense of smell is common among PD patients. In fact, doctors believe that an impaired sense of smell may be an early indicator of PD, and research is under way to use the loss of the sense of smell as a diagnostic tool for early detection of PD. Some PD patients recall losing part of their sense of smell months or years before other major PD symptoms developed.

Urinary Problems/Constipation

Some individuals with PD may have difficulty controlling their bowels and bladder and suffer constipation. As mentioned earlier, malfunctioning neurons in the brain affect smooth muscle movement throughout the body, and this may also affect the function of the digestive system. Also, it's possible that some medications you take may cause constipation. Making changes in diet and exercise and drinking plenty of fluids can often alleviate constipation.

Difficulty Sleeping

Those with PD may experience restless sleep, nightmares, and problems staying asleep at night. As a result, they may feel drowsy during the day. Difficulty sleeping may be a symptom of PD or a side effect of the drugs used to treat symptoms of the disease.

Changes in Facial Expression

PD can cause one to have diminished facial expressions. A person may smile or frown less and facial expressions may become somewhat "masklike." A person with PD may also blink less and appear to stare. These changes are a result of the complex changes that occur in the body as the result of reduced dopamine levels.

Oily/Dry Skin

It is common for people with PD to develop either oily or dry skin, sweat excessively, and be unusually sensitive to feelings of heat or cold. Medication and standard skin treatments can usually alleviate these problems.

Changes in Handwriting

It is not uncommon for patients with PD to notice changes in their handwriting; it often becomes small and crowded. The change in handwriting is a result of not enough dopamine getting to the brain; the resulting disruption in muscle movement affects handwriting.

Stages of PD: How the Disease Progresses

PD affects people differently. In some, the disease progresses quickly. Some patients with PD, however, experience a slower progression. Some people with PD become quite disabled from the symptoms; some individuals with PD experience only minor symptoms.

For most PD patients, there is a subtle "presymptomatic" phase, which may begin four to six years before more obvious symptoms. A person may feel tired or generally unwell. He or she may feel a bit shaky or have trouble getting out of a chair. Other subtle, early symptoms may include:

- Slight weakness in an extremity
- Stiffness in one leg when walking
- Slight trembling
- Mood changes
- Changes in posture
- Decreased sense of smell
- Memory problems
- Dizziness
- Changes in handwriting
- Changes in speech
- Muscle and joint pains

Often the disease begins with a small tremor that comes and goes in one finger. Over time, however, the tremor may become more frequent and spread to the entire arm. Stiffness or rigidity in the arm can follow. Simple tasks such as buttoning clothes may become difficult. With time, the leg on the affected side becomes stiff, harder to move.

In many cases these changes are so subtle or gradual a person doesn't really notice them. Often, family or friends are the first to notice a change in their loved one. As the years pass, the symptoms progress. The tremor and the rigidity may spread to both sides of the body. Movement may become slower. One's facial expression becomes less animated.

Especially in older people, it is easy to see how stiff limbs, slow movement, and a shuffling gait may be confused with normal, age-related changes. Many people with PD and their loved ones dismiss the early symptoms as "old age." Sometimes the fatigue and lack of facial expression lead to an incorrect diagnosis of depression. Because the symptoms often progress slowly over many years, it may take quite some time before they interfere enough to prompt one to seek a medical diagnosis.

Doctors classify PD symptoms by stages. For example, your doctor may say, "You have stage 1 Parkinson's disease." Here's a description of the stages.

Stage 1

- Signs and symptoms appear on only one side of the body.
- Symptoms are mild.
- Symptoms may be inconvenient, but they are not disabling.
- Usually a tremor is present in only one limb.
- Friends and other loved ones notice changes in posture, movement, and facial expression.

Stage 2

- Symptoms appear on both sides of the body.
- Symptoms cause minimal disability.

- Posture and gait are affected.

Stage 3
- Body movements are slowed significantly.
- Symptoms cause moderate to severe problems with normal functioning.

Stage 4
- Symptoms are severe.
- The individual can still walk, but only to a limited extent.
- The patient experiences rigidity and slowness of movement.
- One is no longer able to live alone.

Neurologists include a fifth stage in which the debilitation requires a patient to be confined to a bed or wheelchair. For many patients, early self-help and drug therapy may delay this stage to very late in the disease or even prevent it altogether.

Who Gets PD?

You may be asking, "Why did I get PD?" No one really knows. But you're not alone. Parkinson's disease strikes about two out of a thousand people in the general population and about five per thousand among those fifty and older. It is uncommon, though not unheard of, in children and young adults. PD is equally common among men and women and occurs in all ethnic groups.

About 60,000 new cases are diagnosed annually in the United States alone. At least a million Americans have been diagnosed with Parkinson's disease, and research suggests that there might be twice as many undiagnosed cases. The incidence of PD is expected to double by the year 2030.

More people suffer from PD than from multiple sclerosis, muscular dystrophy, and amyotrophic lateral sclerosis (Lou Gehrig's disease) combined.

What Causes PD?

The precise cause of Parkinson's disease is not known. However, researchers have uncovered clues about the causes. It is clear that a lack of the chemical dopamine in the brain is a major factor. There are other theories about possible causes.

Damage to Nerve Cells

Parkinson's disease is caused by the progressive deterioration of the brain's nerve cells, which produce the chemical dopamine. As mentioned earlier, when production of this chemical is impaired, normal nerve function is disrupted, which in turn affects the coordination of movement. Medical scientists are not sure why degeneration of these nerve cells occurs.

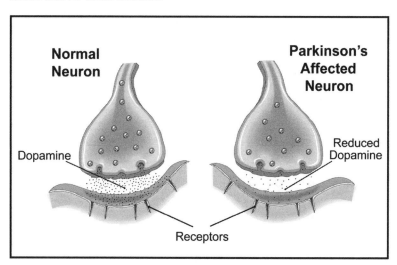

Parkinson's symptoms are caused by the lack of dopamine in the brain. Notice how the damaged nerve cell on the right produces far less dopamine than the normal cell on the left.

Free Radicals

Other causes of PD are certainly possible. Some researchers suggest that *free radicals* (also called *oxidants*) may damage or kill nerve cells and lead to PD. Free radicals are highly unstable molecules produced during the body's normal metabolism. These free radicals cause cell damage only when there are more than the body can handle.

Antioxidants such as vitamins A, C, and E neutralize free radicals. The damage occurs when your intake of antioxidants (from food or supplements) is too low or when your body produces excessive amounts of free radicals due to inflammation, drug or alcohol abuse, smoking, sun damage, or dozens of other factors. Cancer, heart disease, and Parkinson's disease are only a few of the disorders in which free radicals play a role.

Environmental Toxins

Many scientists believe external or internal toxins may destroy the dopamine-messenger nerve cells in the brain. The synthetic drug MPTP is an example of one such external toxin. A potential by-product of synthetically produced "designer drugs," MPTP has been associated with the rapid onset of PD symptoms in some drug abusers.

Similarly, some scientists suggest that drug reactions or exposure to pesticides, carbon monoxide, heavy metals, or toxins in the food supply may also cause damage to the brain cells that produce dopamine.

Accelerated Aging

Another theory proposes that PD symptoms occur when the normal, age-related wearing away of dopamine-producing neurons speeds up. The reason for this accelerated aging is not known.

Genetic Factors

A relatively new theory suggests that the tendency to develop PD may be inherited. Some families have multiple cases of PD, but these are rare. Without an obvious family history, the risk of your offspring developing PD is probably low.

Usage of Certain Drugs

As mentioned, a PD-like state—usually reversible—may be caused by certain drugs. For instance, some tranquilizers *(haloperidol, thioridazine, chlorpromazine)* and drugs used to treat high blood pressure that contain *resperine* may interfere with the dopamine in the brain and cause symptoms of PD. Also, prolonged use of *antipsychotic* (*neuroleptic*) *drugs,* such as those used to treat schizophrenia, may cause a type of Parkinsonism, but it is reversible once the drug is stopped.

How Is PD Diagnosed?

In the early stages, PD may be difficult to diagnose. Early symptoms may be vague and seemingly unrelated. They may mysteriously come and go. As mentioned earlier, PD symptoms may be confused with normal, age-related changes or with symptoms of other disorders, including Huntington's disease, normal pressure hydrocephalis, multisystem atrophy, progressive supernuclear palsy, dementia with Lewy body disease, and Wilson's disease. Some people with hardened, narrowed arteries (*arteriosclerosis*) who have suffered strokes develop PD-like symptoms. In such cases, an accurate diagnosis of PD may prove difficult, especially since there are no blood or lab tests that can definitively diagnose PD.

Diagnosing PD may be difficult even for a neurologist familiar with the disease. Doctors diagnose it with a neurological examination that includes looking at the type and severity of symptoms, especially the three classic PD symptoms: tremors, rigidity, and slowness of movement.

A physician may suggest a trial of anti-Parkinson drugs, usually levodopa. If symptoms improve with the drug, PD is the likely diagnosis. If not, the problem may be caused by something else. The doctor may also want to conduct scans of the brain. Although neither *computed tomography* (CT) nor *magnetic resonance imaging* (MRI) can diagnose PD, these brain-imaging tools can rule out other diseases that may produce PD-like symptoms.

Get a second and even a third opinion, if needed. If only one doctor says you have PD, it is easy to say, "That doctor doesn't know what he's is talking about." But if two or three doctors confirm the diagnosis, PD is harder to deny.

Be realistic about your symptoms. How long have you felt not quite yourself? Make a list of all the symptoms you have noticed. Then read the list over. Do you have any of the "classic" PD symptoms—tremor, slowness of movement, or stiffness?

Ask friends and family for their opinions. What symptoms have they noticed?

Give yourself time. It is difficult to accept that you have a chronic, progressive disease. Take your time. Try to gradually take a new view of things.

A Final Word

Even though the possible symptoms listed in this chapter can be worrisome, remember that not every person with PD develops every symptom listed. And as noted earlier, PD symptoms vary from person to person. The symptoms are slowly progressive from the onset and generally do not become worse suddenly.

Also keep in mind that you can do a lot to cope with PD. Subsequent chapters will discuss how drugs can help. And, as the next chapter will discuss, you can develop ways to cope emotionally.

3

The Emotional Side of Parkinson's Disease

L ong-term, chronic ailments such as PD can disrupt family life, strain marriages, alienate friends and colleagues, and drain hard-earned financial resources. Learning you have PD can be devastating. You may feel angry, guilty, afraid, and resentful. You may deny you have the disease, withdraw, or become depressed. One of the most important things to know is that these feelings and reactions are normal. Most people who have been diagnosed with PD experience some or all of them at one time or another.

There are no right or wrong, good or bad reactions to such devastating news. No one can tell you how to react. Your reaction to the disease and how you cope with it will determine the shape and color of your life, and to a lesser degree, the lives of your loved ones.

Overcoming Denial

PD tends to sneak up on people, coming on imperceptibly in small degrees. Before your diagnosis, you probably knew you were "not quite yourself." You may have dismissed your symptoms, denying anything was seriously wrong for as long as you could.

This reaction is normal and very common. Denial is a form of self-protection. We never want to admit something is seriously wrong. Before your diagnosis, you probably found yourself torn between denial of any problem and fear and worry about what the problem might be. As your symptoms progressed and you experienced more physical limitations, the mental strain and worry probably became even more severe.

If you're like most people, you find the diagnosis of PD both a shock and something of a relief. You have just been told that you have a progressive, disabling disease. Yet there is some relief in at last being able to put a name to your vague symptoms.

Suddenly, however, your future looks uncertain. Questions fill your mind: What will I be able to do? Is it possible to continue working? Can I still function as a parent or partner? What kind of medical bills will I have to deal with?

It is not uncommon to refuse to accept a PD diagnosis. Unfortunately, denial expends a great deal of energy and causes anxiety. Trying to hide your symptoms may cause you embarrassment and isolation. As long as you deny the disease, you are its unwitting victim. The sooner you accept your condition, the sooner you can begin coping with it and living your life.

Conquering Unfounded Fears

You may have seen friends, relatives, or acquaintances who suffered from PD before there were effective medications such as *levodopa* (l-dopa), when PD was more disabling and less treatable than it is today. Fortunately, many of the symptoms of PD can now be successfully treated with medications.

19

Here are several ways to combat unfounded fears and to prevent your imagination from causing you undue distress:

Find a doctor you can work with. Look for someone who will talk with you about your fears and concerns. *Learn all you can about the disease.* Read books. Look up information on Web sites that post reliable information. *Talk about your fears with your doctor, your family, and supportive friends.* It helps to "air" your fears. When you bring them into the light, they appear less overwhelming.

Join a PD support group. Aside from providing camaraderie and moral support, members of such groups can give information about the latest treatments, referrals to physicians, and practical tips on how to cope.

Talk with a mental-health professional. If you've followed all these suggestions and still feel overwhelmed, talk with a neuropsychologist or another mental-health professional.

Regaining a Sense of Control

A common reaction to a diagnosis of PD is "Why me?" Suddenly your life seems dangerously out of control. As much as you might try to manage your life, there are times when you are helpless. You can't do anything about a slick, icy patch on the road; a mechanical failure on an airplane you're flying; or the fact that the dopamine in your brain is depleted.

Seeing yourself as a victim saps your energy and motivation and makes you feel needlessly dependent on others. The good news is you can regain a sense of control in your life.

Although you can't do anything about having PD, there is plenty you can do about how it affects your life.

Learning about PD can quiet your fears as well as renew your sense of independence. To regain your equilibrium, consider the following:

Become an active participant in your health care. Don't just passively accept what your doctor says. Ask questions. If you don't understand, ask questions until you do. Offer suggestions.

Stay as independent as possible. Some people react to chronic illness by becoming increasingly dependent on others. Eventually, these folks may become totally helpless, not from the disease itself but from their emotional reactions to it. Instead, do as much for yourself as you can, asking for help only when you really need it.

Make a plan for yourself. Work closely with your doctor to develop an effective treatment plan. Make a list of all the things you can do to help yourself, such as exercising, eating right, managing stress, and taking your medicine on time.

Reclaiming a Sense of Self

"Who am I?" you may wonder. Be assured that you are more than your disease. You may not be able to perform daily activities to the same degree as before your PD diagnosis, but you are still a valuable individual. Here are some tips for bolstering your internal defenses and reclaiming a strong sense of self.

Learn to accept help when you really need it. It is difficult to be dependent on others, but your condition will make you unable to do certain things. You *will* need help. Learn to accept this increased level of dependence without losing your dignity.

Learn to cope with negative responses from others. Sometimes, you will have to deal with rudeness or insensitivity from others, especially strangers. If people stare or show hostility, pity, or rejection, chalk it up to their igno-rance about this complex disease.

Talk with others about how they cope. Others with chronic diseases have walked the same road and know how it feels. Talking and sharing feelings, thoughts, and ideas with them can help you feel less alone and less differ-ent.

Recall your past successes. This suggestion doesn't mean dwelling on the past or grieving for what was. Just keep in mind your past contributions, honors, and achieve-ments. Those memories can bolster your spirits when you are feeling down.

Focus on small victories. It's not the huge successes that count over time, but dozens of small ones. Set goals and keep track of your successes. Consider keeping a writ-ten or taped journal of your victories and review it often to keep your spirits up.

Avoid lashing out. Sometimes you will feel angry about your disease. Avoid taking out your anger on others, especially loved ones and caregivers.

Avoid destructive behaviors. Some people turn to drugs and alcohol to numb the pain of difficult challenges such as chronic illness. These "fixes" are only temporary and ultimately will make your disease more difficult to deal with.

Overcoming Depression

Depression is common among people with PD, affect-ing about half of those with the disease. Depression is dif-ferent from and more serious than "the blues" that most of us feel from time to time. The symptoms of depression include:

- Depressed mood

- Diminished interest or loss of pleasure in activities
- Weight loss when not dieting or weight gain
- Inability to sleep or oversleeping
- Restlessness (agitation) or slowing down so that it is noticeable to others
- Fatigue or loss of energy
- Feelings of worthlessness
- Diminished ability to think or concentrate
- Recurrent thoughts of suicide or death

If you experience several of these symptoms for two weeks or longer, you are likely depressed. Though most people with PD experience only mild depression, a few suffer moderate or even severe depression.

Depression may be caused by biochemical changes in the brains of some people with PD. Studies have revealed that those who suffer from depression have reduced levels of *serotonin*, a brain chemical believed to play a major role in the regulation of mood. Doctors call this biochemical imbalance in the brain *endogenous depression*, which can be life threatening if not treated.

Medications used to treat PD may also cause depression. Usually, depression caused by PD medications starts with anxiety, restlessness, or worry in the first two weeks after beginning the drug treatment. This period may be followed by sleeplessness, mood swings, or both for several weeks. Symptoms usually peak after five or six weeks as the body adapts to the medication and the depression begins to lift. If you believe your depression is related to the medications you are taking, talk with your doctor. Perhaps your prescription or dosage can be changed.

Because some of the symptoms of depression—fatigue, slow movement, insomnia, difficulty concentrating—are also PD symptoms, PD-related depression is often confused or misdiagnosed. In the early stages, depression might mask PD symptoms. Later on, PD symptoms may hide depression.

If you have symptoms of depression, it is important to have them treated. Your doctor can prescribe antidepressant medication, which may also alleviate other PD symptoms. Here are other suggestions that can lift your spirits:

Get active. Physical activity releases *endorphins*, the body's own natural mood elevators. If you cannot accomplish a task because you're tired or "off," do something else. The key is to remain as physically and mentally active as possible.

Identify your goals. To keep depressive feelings from overwhelming you, set small, specific goals that are realistic and attainable. Establish a time frame for each goal. Set goals in all areas of your life: physical activity, employment, social activities, spiritual growth, and recreational activities, such as crafts, that will help tune your motor skills. Your list of goals may look something like this:

- Exercise at least fifteen minutes every day.
- Attend a PD support group once a week.
- Take a class on the Internet this month.

Avoid self-criticism. It's easy to be critical of yourself when you are feeling depressed. When you hear that inner voice giving negative messages such as "I'm too slow" or "I used to be able to do this, but now I can't," refocus attention on accomplishments. Replace negative messages with positive ones, such as "I do my job well," "I'm an excellent parent," or "I have a good relationship with my family."

Stay connected with others. It's not unusual for people in the early stages of PD to feel embarrassed about their symptoms, especially tremors. When it's difficult or awkward for you to move around, you might feel uncomfortable in social situations. To avoid embarrassment, you may withdraw from others and pass up your usual social and recreational activities.

Isolation only intensifies your depression. Staying connected is vitally important to your mental and emotional health. Seize opportunities to interact with other people by participating in church activities, entertaining, taking classes, visiting friends, volunteering, and attending support-group meetings.

Talk about your feelings. Share your thoughts, feelings, fears, concerns, hopes, and dreams with friends and loved ones. Don't be afraid to talk about your loneliness, embarrassment, anger, and frustration. You may be surprised to learn how sharing your inner feelings can deepen your relationships.

Try counseling. If these strategies don't provide enough relief, consider talking with a mental-health counselor for additional support.

Reducing Stress

Stress can often make PD symptoms, especially tremors, worse. Although researchers have ruled out stress as a cause of PD, stress can trigger symptoms or magnify them. It is important to effectively manage stress.

Identify sources of stress. Different things are stressful to different people. Even pleasant situations may be stressful. For many with PD, especially those newly diagnosed, social events may cause anxiety and worsen symptoms, resulting in even more stress. Rather than refusing to socialize and becoming isolated, evaluate social situations and decide how you can make changes to reduce the stress. Make a list of those things that cause you stress.

Make and follow through on a stress-reduction plan. For example, maybe the last time you dined with friends, several pieces of your lunch ended up on the floor because you had difficulty cutting the meat. You felt humiliated and embarrassed, vowing to decline such invitations in the future.

Instead, ask yourself, "How could I do this differently? How could I accommodate my condition and still enjoy lunching with my friends?" Possible solutions include ordering a dish that does not require the fine motor skills needed to cut meat, asking your companion to cut your meat, and asking your server to cut your portion into bite-size pieces before bringing it to the table.

Adjust your expectations. Pushing yourself to perform mentally and physically exactly as you once did may bring on undue anxiety.

Reprioritize. A serious illness forces you to reevaluate your life. What's really important to you? Is it closing one more sale or spending more time with your granddaughter? Is it earning more money or volunteering for a cause you feel passionate about? Only you can decide what's most important.

This kind of self-examination may result in your changing jobs or easing up on your housekeeping standards. Your new priorities may bring you closer to your true self and what makes you happy.

Set goals. Make your goals realistic and attainable but also challenging, so that they make you "stretch" just a bit. Take time to set goals in all areas of your life: social, spiritual, physical, financial, and so on. Establish weekly goals and longer-term goals.

Plan your time so as to avoid stressful deadlines. Many of us are caught in a time crunch. We often rush, barely getting to appointments on time. Allow more time for everything. Whenever possible, set approximate times for appointments so that if you're running behind you won't be late.

Get plenty of sleep. Plan your schedule whenever possible so that you get extra rest after a particularly busy day. If your lifestyle allows it, take a refreshing nap every afternoon. Research has shown that short afternoon naps (less than forty-five minutes) can make you more relaxed, refreshed, and alert.

Limit caffeine. It can make you jittery. Coffee, black tea, cola, and other beverages often contain caffeine, as does chocolate. Drink decaf varieties or limit yourself to one caffeinated cup a day. Avoid drinking caffeinated beverages before retiring for the night.

Get organized. Develop systems to help you find things easily. Put items in the same place every day. For instance, putting your keys, purse, or wallet in a designated place will spare you the anxiety of not being able to find them, especially when you're rushed.

Ask for help. As mentioned, no one likes to feel dependent. But you will need to ask family and friends for assistance with some activities. Asking for aid from others not only allows you to be vulnerable and open, it allows them to give you the gift of help. At first it may be difficult, but over time such interdependence can bring people closer together.

Practice deep breathing. Sit quietly with your eyes closed. To the count of four, breathe in deeply, filling your lungs and your abdomen. Then slowly release it. Repeat for five or six breaths.

Progressively relax. Sit or lie in a quiet place where you won't be disturbed. Starting at your head, tense and then release groups of muscles. Work down your entire body, progressively tensing and releasing muscles. Once you've tensed and released all the way to your feet, sit or lie quietly for several minutes.

Meditate. Take a meditation class. Or try this simple meditation technique: Sit quietly with your eyes closed, breathing normally. Each time you inhale, think the word "one" (or "peace," "calm," or "om"). As thoughts come up, let them go and gently refocus on your word and your breathing. Continue for ten to fifteen minutes. At first, you may be bothered by many thoughts, or so-called "monkey mind." Don't worry. With practice, you will find that you are better able to quiet your mind and enjoy the peaceful silence. Take a meditation break in the morning and in the early evening, or whenever you are feeling tired or overwhelmed.

Practice yoga. Yoga can calm your mind and keep your body more limber. Many postures involve gentle stretching, strengthening, and deep breathing.

Explore biofeedback. This exercise involves learning to control your own body functions with visual or auditory stimulation. You will first have to learn the techniques from a physician or a biofeedback technician. Once you have learned them, however, you will undoubtedly feel more in control of your stress level and your body.

Relax with guided imagery. Hundreds of recordings are available for purchase or loan from the library that combine relaxing sounds or music with instructions for an imaginary "trip." For instance, guided imagery might involve visualizing yourself walking by the sea on a beautiful, cloudless day and feeling the wind caress your skin, or lying in a green meadow where you can smell the flowers, hear the gentle twitter of birds, and feel the sun warming your body. Once you become accustomed to using these recordings, you will be able to visualize on your own and take a little "mental vacation" whenever the need arises.

Telling Others about Your Disease

Telling others about your PD may cause anxiety and stress. When should you tell others? Whom should you tell? Should you tell your employer? What about your children or grandchildren? How much should you tell?

There are no right or wrong answers to these questions. Some people opt to tell everyone they know to avoid questions and curious looks. Others choose to tell only those closest to them until symptoms become evident. You must find your own answers to these questions.

One thing is certain. Attempting to hide your disease, especially as symptoms worsen, will make you more anxious. Anxiety, in turn, may worsen your symptoms. Medical experts have found that those who are able to accept their disease and tell others about it cope best.

Keep in mind that PD affects not only you but all those close to you. Effectively coping with and treating PD requires the assistance, understanding, and cooperation of everyone in your social network. Keeping it a secret just makes it harder to begin the process of coming to terms with your disease. Below are general tips about telling family, friends, coworkers, acquaintances, employers, and others about your condition:

Be direct and honest. Once you decide who to tell, there's no use trying to sugarcoat the situation. At work, it's a good idea to talk with your supervisor before telling coworkers.

Don't wait too long. If your symptoms are noticeable, friends and coworkers will naturally wonder what's wrong and will probably come up with an incorrect "diagnosis."

Let people know how they can help, especially as your needs change.

Help others learn about PD. Some people, especially those who are close to you, may need to learn more about PD. Finding out about the disease can reassure them that there are many people with PD who are living full and active lives. An abundance of literature is available online or in printed form from a variety of sources, including the national PD organizations listed in the Resource section of this book. You'll also find information on the Internet and at the library.

Talking with Your Partner

When you have a chronic illness, your partner is affected almost as much as you are. If he or she isn't present when you receive your PD diagnosis, it's important that you share the information as soon as possible.

Any long-term illness can strain a marriage or long-term relationship to the breaking point. If the relationship is already on shaky ground, a diagnosis of Parkinson's disease may be the final blow. Your partner may not be able or willing to endure the realities of long-term illness. Common reactions may include going into denial; feeling angry or resentful that major aspects of the relationship may change, including traditional roles; and becoming fearful and overprotective, always wanting to "take care" of you. Although these responses are perfectly normal and quite common, none is productive.

If you're fortunate enough to have a stable, loving relationship, the diagnosis of PD will test but not destroy your partnership. Instead, over time, it may bring you closer together.

Facing your partner's reactions is one of the most difficult aspects of PD. Nevertheless, it is important not to let your mate's responses aggravate your symptoms. Here are some strategies for helping your mate cope:

Be honest about your condition. Don't soft-pedal your prognosis to spare your partner. Likewise, don't try to make it seem more serious than it is. You are in this together, so both of you deserve to be fully and honestly informed.

Accept his or her reactions. Remember, there are no "right" ways for a partner to respond to this kind of life-changing news.

Reassure. Let your mate know that, with treatment, most people with PD live long and productive lives and that most, if not all, symptoms can be controlled.

Remain as independent as possible. Be realistic: Ask for help when you need it, but don't become overly dependent. Caregiving is difficult. Your partner has enough to do without your making excessive demands.

Encourage your mate to fully participate with your health care team. This involvement will help both of you feel that you're in it together.

Learn about the disease together. Both partners should gather materials about PD and learn as much as possible about the disease.

Encourage your partner to attend caregiver support groups. Many communities offer support groups for partner-caregivers in which they can talk about their feelings, get practical tips for coping, and feel less alone.

Support your partner's outside interests and relationships. It is important for your mate to develop and maintain personal and recreational interests such as community and religious activities, sports, friendships, and classes. Your mate will feel less stressed and will be a better caregiver if he or she isn't entirely absorbed by you and your illness.

Honestly discuss your finances. One of the biggest fears a partner faces when the other person becomes ill is the loss of income. Sit down and take a realistic look at your financial situation. Review your health insurance. Develop a realistic budget. Can you cut some expenses to save money? If needed, check out governmental sources of financial assistance.

Assess your support system. Who else in your circle of family and friends can you count on for help? Full-time partner-caregivers need help and respite. If your partner can't drive you to the doctor, who else can?

Talk, talk, talk. Close communication is a key component to coping effectively with PD and maintaining a harmonious relationship. Good communication can make the difference between a partnership that weathers the storm and one that founders.

Talking with Children

At some point children, too, need to be told. Here are some tips for talking with children about your disease.

Use age-appropriate language. Too much or too little information given in a way that feels scary or threatening may stimulate a child's fantasies and fears. To a young child you might say, "Grandmother has a sickness that makes her hands shake." To a teenager you might say, "I have a nerve problem that makes my hands tremble." Don't speculate about what the future holds. As the condition progresses, you may need to give more information.

Encourage children to ask questions. Kids are wonderful at asking direct questions, especially if you let them know it's all right to talk about your condition. "Why don't you stand up straight, Grandpa?" "Why don't you smile, Mommy?" "Why is your voice so soft, Aunt Mary?"

Let children share their concerns. Fears that are suppressed may grow out of proportion. Create an open atmosphere that allows children to express their fears, anxieties, and concerns about your condition.

Reassure. Let children know that your condition isn't fatal and that it isn't contagious. Often, children are afraid they might "catch" others' health problems. Inform older children about how most evidence suggests that PD is not an inherited disease. Also reassure them that you didn't get the disease because of anything they or anyone else did or did not do.

Keep the tone light and conversational. If you cry or let your anxiety show, children may worry unnecessarily. Approaching PD calmly and matter-of-factly will help them keep things in perspective. The more accepting you are of your condition, the more accepting children will be.

Use humor. Humor can often make difficult situations tolerable. Don't use humor to mask reality or hide your real feelings, because children will know you aren't being genuine. But when you can laugh at yourself and your condition, it makes the situation easier to handle.

Telling Your Employer

Some people are diagnosed with PD after they've retired, so telling an employer is not an issue. However, other people are still employed when they are diagnosed. "Should I tell my employer?" is a question often asked by people newly diagnosed with PD. Perhaps a more realistic question is, "When should I tell my employer?"

Unfortunately, there is no clear-cut answer. Each situation is different. The kind of job you have will affect when you will need to tell your boss. For instance, an airline pilot or a brain surgeon with Parkinson's disease will likely have to tell his or her employer sooner than someone who sells insurance. How rapidly your disease progresses and how well your symptoms can be controlled with medications will also affect when you tell your employer—as will the kind of relationship you have with your supervisor and the organization.

No one can predict the outcome of informing an employer. Your supervisor might be flexible about your doctor's appointments and make accommodations in your work environment to make your job easier. Other employers are less empathetic. You may be reassigned to other job duties or be pressured into early retirement.

Remember, PD is a disability. You are protected under federal law from being fired solely because you have PD, although it may prove difficult and costly to win such a case in court. Here are some guidelines to consider before talking with your employer:

- Discuss your work situation and any workplace limitations openly with your doctors.

- Ask your doctors about accommodations that might make it possible for you to continue being productive in your job.

- Make a list of the pros and cons of telling your employer. Realistically look at your situation and ask yourself, "Can I still do this job and do it well?"

- Have some suggestions for accommodation to offer your employer. Perhaps, like many telecommuters today, you can work out of your home.

Adapting to Changing Roles and Finding Focus

PD will invariably change your roles both at home and at work. It will likely change how you view yourself, too. It's important to keep in mind that you are not your disease. You happen to be a person with PD. Your condition is simply a part of who you are.

At home, you may no longer be able to perform your usual tasks and this could affect how you feel about yourself. You may find your partner and children taking on responsibilities—such as driving, paying bills, making decisions, and planning the social calendar—that you used to do yourself or together.

For some people, nothing represents independence like the automobile. However, the changes in motor and concentration skills make it important for people with PD to be realistic about their ability to continue driving. Some patients with PD willingly give up their driver's license. Others are adamant about retaining this symbol of their independence. At some point, it will be crucial to have your driving skills assessed by a professional driving instructor to determine whether it is still safe for you to drive.

In this chapter, we have dealt primarily with coping with losses. But what are you going to put in place of those losses? It's vitally important that you reprioritize, finding new focus and meaning in your life.

For many of us, work defines who we are. We don't say, "I'm a loving, loyal person." Instead we say, "I'm a doctor (or lawyer, secretary, teacher, writer)." When that work role changes or disappears, we may find ourselves at a loss.

Not everyone with PD has to give up his or her profession. Many can still work effectively. If you can still perform your job with competence, stay with it as long as possible. If changes in your physical and mental capabilities make it difficult to continue in your occupation, look for ways to change your job or make accommodations that might enable you to keep working. Using computers, faxes, cell phones, and other technological devices, perhaps you can work out of your home, as mentioned earlier.

If your current job becomes too difficult, consider another vocation. Take a look at your experience and skills. How can you put them to work in another capacity? Perhaps you can work as a consultant, start your own business, or find a less demanding part-time job. The point is to stay productive and to contribute for as long as you are able.

Not everyone can or wants to continue working. Many people are near or at retirement age when they develop PD and would rather engage in other pursuits. That's fine, too, as long as those pursuits provide a sense of focus, purpose, fulfillment, and accomplishment. Perhaps you can become involved in church, community, or volunteer activities, thereby shifting your focus from personal problems to helping others. Or for a rewarding experience, consider taking a class in an area of interest or teaching a class to adults or children.

4

Your Doctor as Partner

When you have a chronic disease such as Parkinson's disease, a good relationship with your doctors is vital. After all, you and your doctors will likely deal with this disease together for years to come.

Many of us grew up believing that doctors are somehow magical, that their advice is always right, and that a patient's role is simply to do exactly as the doctor instructs, no questions asked. Times have changed. The demands of a complicated and challenging disease such as PD require that you establish and maintain a strong partnership with your doctors. Each of you will bring information and expertise to the partnership.

Your doctors and other professionals on your health care team will provide the medical and clinical expertise. You will bring expertise about yourself—how you feel both physically and emotionally and how those feelings change over time. As a partner in your health care, you have the right to question or reject any medication or surgical procedure your doctor recommends. You also have the right to a second opinion. You and your doctors must cooperatively make decisions about your care. A strong partnership will help ensure that you get the best treatment for your condition.

Your Health Care Team

People with PD usually have at least two doctors: a primary-care physician and a neurologist. A *primary-care physician* is your "regular" doctor, your family physician. Usually a primary-care physician is an internist, a family practitioner, or a general practitioner.

Your primary-care physician will probably refer you to a specialist, the neurologist. Depending on your condition and your medical insurance plan, your primary-care physician may follow and treat your disease, as well as any other health problems as they come up. Your insurance plan may allow you to see a neurologist or other specialist only periodically.

A *neurologist* is a doctor who has specialized training in disorders and treatment of the nervous system. Since PD is a nervous-system disorder, it is important that you be evaluated by a neurologist. Ideally, your neurologist should make or confirm the diagnosis of PD, recommend symptomatic treatment, and monitor treatment.

Neurologists, like many other physicians, often have different interests and experience. Some neurologists continue their training in a specialized area now termed "movement disorders"—that is, diseases that have movements as their symptoms. Some even go on to do clinical and research work in university-based PD research centers. If your community has one of these research centers, you will find qualified neurologists there. Wherever you live, look for a neurologist who has interest, training, and experience in treating patients with PD.

Depending on your symptoms, you may need other specialized treatment. For instance, some people with PD experience mental disturbances—difficult thoughts, feelings, and behaviors as well as memory losses. A *psychia-*

trist, a medical doctor with special training in mental health, can diagnose and treat mental disorders. He or she may use psychotherapy, marital and family counseling, and medications to help with PD-related mental-health issues. A psychiatrist may see you initially and then refer you to another mental-health provider, such as a *clinical psychologist* or a *social worker,* for longer-term treatment. Often, families with loved ones who have PD have a whole range of needs, including financial, emotional, and social. A social worker is trained in family and marital therapy and can help you access other community services as well. (Such providers are often less expensive than psychiatrists. Whom you see may depend on your health insurance policy.)

If you have problems with self-care, employment, or leisure activities, your doctor may refer you to an *occupational therapist.* This professional can help you choose adaptation equipment to safely cope with many of your symptoms and make life easier.

A *physical therapist* can help you deal with mobility, posture, and balance problems. He or she is trained to assess such physical problems and prescribe appropriate exercises. In addition, a physical therapist can help you determine which leisure physical activities are best for you.

A *speech therapist* helps with oral communication and swallowing difficulties.

A *massage therapist* can provide short-term help for stiff muscles and rigidity. Check your health plan to determine whether such services are covered.

If you need help with dietary matters, a *dietitian* can help. He or she can help you plan a healthy diet and devise ways to prepare meals that accommodate your limitations.

Your *pharmacist* can be an important part of your health care team because pharmacists do more than just dispense medications. He or she can answer your questions about medications, keep track of potentially dangerous drug interactions, and advise you on supplements and over-the-counter medications. For best results, use only one pharmacy—preferably one that has a computer system for tracking all the drugs you're taking. In addition, select a pharmacist who will take the time to carefully explain your medications and answer your questions.

Choosing the Right Doctor

A first step in taking an active role in your health care is to choose the right doctor and other members of your health care team. With a long-term disease such as PD, it's especially important that you and your health care team develop a special bond. It's essential to have the right "fit," so that you can talk honestly and openly with your physician and other health care team members. They must demonstrate the time, energy, personality, and expertise to provide you with the best care. You must be able to trust that the advice your health care professionals give you is entirely in your best interest.

Where do you find the right doctor and other specialists who can help you with your condition? Unless your insurance company is very restrictive, you may seek referrals from:

- Friends, relatives, coworkers, and acquaintances
- Other doctors, nurses, and pharmacists
- PD support groups
- A national PD Foundation office
- Area hospitals or medical schools
- State or county medical associations (ask for a list of board-certified neurologists)

- Area PD research centers
- Your insurance company's preferred-provider list

A Word about HMOs

Since the introduction of health maintenance organizations (HMOs), choosing the right doctor has become a bit more complicated. HMOs have changed the way we select our health care providers. Under most HMO plans, you must see a primary-care doctor before you can be referred to a specialist such as a neurologist. Some plans allow such a referral only under special circumstances. You might also have to select from the plan's list of preferred providers. If you choose a doctor not on the preferred-provider list, your insurance will likely not cover the cost unless preapproved by the administrator of your plan.

However, even under HMO plans, you have choices. Ask friends and coworkers who have the same insurance plan for recommendations. If you are not satisfied with the first doctor you see on your HMO's list, find another preferred provider. Having a particular type of insurance doesn't mean that you must see a doctor with whom you're not comfortable.

If your primary-care doctor seems hesitant to refer you to a specialist, be assertive. Tell him or her it's time you saw a neurologist. As mentioned earlier, make sure the specialist is covered under your plan.

What makes a good doctor or other health care specialist? For some patients, a doctor's promptness is important. For others, it's more important that the doctor or specialist be personable. Only you can decide what's critical for you in your healthcare team. Take a moment to review the list below. Then make your own list and use it to select your healthcare team.

A Checklist for Evaluating
the Right Health-Care Team

___Are you comfortable with this doctor/specialist? Does his or her personality "fit" with yours?

___Do you feel you could openly discuss all your concerns and feelings with this health care provider, even sensitive or potentially embarrassing subjects such as sexual or emotional problems?

___Do you feel you could ask this health care provider even "silly" questions?

___Does this provider listen well and answer all your questions in language you can understand?

___If you don't understand something, is he or she willing to take the time to translate complex medical jargon? Is he or she willing to use visual aids to further your understanding?

___Does this health care provider welcome your partner (or other patient advocate) as an active participant in your treatment?

___Does he or she allow enough time for you during office visits so that you don't feel rushed?

___Does he or she seem interested in you and your condition?

___Is this person empathetic, able to put himself or herself in your shoes?

___Is he or she on time?

___Does this provider have experience treating PD patients? Special training?

___Does this provider, doctor or pharmacist, thoroughly explain your medications—how they work, what they're supposed to do, when and how to take them, side effects to watch out for, and what to do if you miss a dose?

____Does your health care professional educate you about PD during your visits? Does he or she give you printed materials and information about books and Web sites that might be helpful?

____Is he or she willing to talk with you about alternative or experimental treatments?

____Does your provider explain self-help strategies, such as exercise and diet?

____Is this doctor willing to refer you to the proper specialists as needed?

____Is he or she available in emergencies? Has he or she explained what you should do in an emergency?

____Is your health care professional readily available by phone or e-mail?

____Does he or she return your phone calls or answer your e-mail promptly?

Communicating with Your Health-Care Team

Good communication is a key component to a strong partnership with your doctor and other members of your health care team. When you are first diagnosed and as your disease progresses, you will have many questions.

Communication is a two-way street. You must give your providers honest, straightforward information about your condition, your feelings, and your ability to stick with your treatment plan. Let them know

- how well your medications are working.
- if you experience any side effects from the drugs.

- about strategies you have discovered that make your medications or other parts of your treatment plan more effective.
- about any new symptoms you may have experienced.
- if you are planning to travel overseas.
- about any other problems you are having with your treatment plan.

Getting the Most from Your Office Visits

You will want to get the most from every visit with your doctors. Why? PD progresses slowly, so you will likely see your doctors only periodically. During visits, your doctor will probably perform a physical exam and specific physical tests to check your progress. He or she will want to observe you walking and check your manual dexterity. Occasionally, he or she will conduct laboratory tests to monitor your medications. Here are some tips for getting the most from your office visits:

Prioritize your visits. Know what you want to accomplish before you go to the doctor. Perhaps you want the doctor to adjust your medication dosage or talk about ways to cope with new, troubling symptoms. Plan ahead. Make a list of questions and concerns you have and take it with you into the exam room. Be well prepared.

Don't waste time. Keep in mind that your doctor sees many patients. He or she has only a limited amount of time to spend with you. This is especially true under many HMO plans. Your time is valuable, too. Don't waste time on unrelated conversations or chitchat.

Invite your patient advocate. Ask your partner or a close family member, friend, or caregiver to accompany you to the doctor's office. This person may act as your patient advocate, helping you ask questions, giving additional information to the doctor, taking notes, and otherwise acting in your interest. It is especially important to have a patient advocate if you feel shy or intimidated about talking with the doctor or asking questions. If you prefer, your patient advocate may even accompany you into the exam room and into the doctor's office after the exam.

Take notes. It's difficult to remember everything the doctor says. Don't be afraid to make notes while the doctor is talking. You might ask your patient advocate to do this for you or take a tape recorder and record your conversation.

Be honest. Your doctor can help only if he or she has complete and honest information about your condition, your symptoms, and your compliance with your treatment program. Sometimes it's difficult to talk about topics such as sexual dysfunction or to discuss your feelings, but the more candid you are, the better your doctor can plan your treatment.

Be informed. Learn as much as you can from reading, talking with others about PD, and discussing your concerns with your doctor. Be prepared to ask your doctor about new procedures and medications for treating PD. You may wish to subscribe to any of several newsletters dedicated to keeping people with PD up to date about new developments in treatment and research. Such newsletters are available from PD foundations and organizations listed in Resources at the back of this book.

The Case for Patient Advocates

If you asked most people, "Do you want or need a patient advocate?" they would likely say no. We're not used to asking for help, especially the kind of intimate help a patient advocate provides. Many people are embarrassed about having someone else in the exam room. They believe that they can speak for themselves.

As a patient, however, you are not in a good position to act as your own advocate. The nature of PD can make it difficult to make good decisions on your own. In addition, strong emotions and mood swings make it harder to act in a rational, objective manner.

A well-informed partner, family member, friend, or caregiver who knows your history, your needs, and your desires is in the best position to help you help yourself and receive the best treatment possible.

5

Drug Treatment for Parkinson's Disease

The right medications can give you relief from the symptoms of PD. However, there is no one-size-fits-all drug treatment for PD. Just as people vary widely with PD symptoms, they also vary in their responses to drug treatment. Some people do very well with a particular drug. Others may not be able to tolerate a drug, or find that the drug does little to relieve their symptoms. It's important to work closely with your doctor, letting him or her know how you are reacting to and tolerating particular drugs and dosages. Together you can find the right combination of medications for your PD management.

Since PD is a progressive disease, you will likely take different drugs at different stages. In the early stages, doctors often begin treatment with one or more of the less-powerful drugs. Being an informed consumer helps you be a compliant patient. This chapter will help you become familiar with PD drugs, their benefits, and their potential side effects.

Levodopa: The Gold Standard of PD Therapy

Development of the drug *levodopa* or *l-dopa*, which is the treatment of choice today, was a major breakthrough in treating PD symptoms. Levodopa enters the brain and is converted to *dopamine*, the brain chemical lacking in people with PD. The brain can't directly absorb dopamine itself because the chemical can't cross the *blood-brain barrier*, an intricate network of fine blood vessels and cells that filter blood before it reaches the brain.

Levodopa, however, *can* pass through the blood-brain barrier, and enzymes then convert it into dopamine. Levodopa can help you enjoy a relatively normal, active, and productive life for many years. It may dramatically reduce muscle stiffness, tremor, bradykinesia, walking impairment, *hypomimia* (masklike facial expression), memory loss, depression, excessive salivation, and changes in skin texture. It usually allows PD patients to write and speak more clearly, remain more alert, swallow more easily, sleep more soundly, and generally experience an improved sense of overall well-being.

Combining Levodopa with Other Drugs

Levodopa is often combined with a second drug, *carbidopa,* which keeps levodopa from "breaking down" before it reaches the brain. Carbidopa also can reduce levodopa side effects such as nausea, vomiting, abdominal distress, and heart problems.

Sinemet is the brand name for combined carbidopa and levodopa. This drug also comes in a slow-release form, Sinemet CR. The slow-release variety requires fewer repeat doses. However, Sinemet CR can be difficult to absorb in the gastrointestinal tract. Sinemet is usually started in small doses. Then, over time, your doctor adjusts the dosage until the best clinical response is achieved. Even after a therapeutic dose is reached, it may take two or three months to enjoy carbidopa/levodopa's full benefit.

The drug *Stalevo* contains *entacapone (Comtan)* as well as carbidopa and levodopa. Like carbidopa, entacapone works by blocking an enzyme that interferes with the brain's absorption of levodopa. Tests have shown that, compared to Sinemet, Stalevo adds almost an hour and a half of symptom relief each day.

Getting the Most from Levodopa

Take medications exactly on time. You need to follow a strict schedule to prevent or reduce "off" times, when the drug isn't working.

Keep a dose with you. Carry your dose pack with you at all times. (Make sure it is out of the reach of children.) If you get stuck in traffic or are otherwise delayed, you'll still be able to take your dose on time.

Develop a reminder system. Calendars, check-off lists, and alarms can remind you when to take your medication. Some dose packs have alarms that can be set to go off at the right time. Ask your doctor about chewing your tablets if you've missed a dose by an hour or less. It may give you faster relief.

Don't try to make up for missed doses. If you've missed a dose by a few hours, don't take a double dose. It will only increase side effects. Take your regular dose and get back on your schedule.

For maximum absorption, take Sinemet sixty minutes before or after meals. Food in the stomach slows absorption and prevents the maximum amount of levodopa from getting to the brain.

Possible Food and Drug Interactions

Levodopa is a type of *amino acid*. Your bloodstream can transport only a limited amount of amino acid at a time. The more protein you take in, the more amino acid will be circulating in your blood, interfering with the absorption of levodopa.

Some researchers believe the "wearing-off" and "on-off" effects of PD therapy may be caused or worsened by too much protein in the diet. Protein is an essential nutrient, however, so monitor the amount of protein you take in and, as mentioned, separate the timing of your dose and your protein intake by at least an hour.

Talk to your physician about your diet. Special low-protein diets have been developed for people taking levodopa because protein may interfere with the absorption of the drug. Anything that delays the drug from entering the bloodstream will also decrease the amount of the drug that reaches the brain.

Also, consider talking with a dietician who has worked with other PD patients. He or she can help you find a way to make sure you're getting enough protein, but not so much that it interferes with levodopa's effectiveness.

Finally, talk to your physician about other drugs you're taking. Some antidepressants, antipsychotics, antinausea medications, and blood pressure medications can affect dopamine levels and cause possible adverse reactions.

Potential Side Effects of Levodopa

The wearing-off effect. One problem for many people on levodopa therapy is the wearing-off effect. With prolonged use, the drug becomes effective for shorter periods of time. Your symptoms may return before your next scheduled dose—which is unlikely to bring immediate relief, because it takes a while for the brain to absorb the drug. To delay the wearing-off effect, doctors try to keep the levodopa dose as low as possible while still keeping symptoms in check.

On-off and freezing episodes. Eventually, about 30 percent of PD patients experience "on-off" attacks or "freezing"—becoming immobile. Experts believe this occurs because over time dopamine receptors in the brain disappear or lose their ability to take in the dopamine delivered by the levodopa. Your physician may adjust dosages of your medications to help control these symptoms.

Dyskinesia. Another problem with long-term use of levodopa is *dyskinesia*—involuntary nodding, jerking, or twitching, which may be fast or slow, mild or severe. Controlling this disturbing symptom, when severe, can be difficult; again, it requires patience, knowledge, and, often, the skill of a neurologist who can find the right balance of medications.

Nausea. If nausea is a problem, especially in the morning, try eating a few crackers or drinking a glass of juice with your dose.

Other side effects are usually temporary, but you should report them to your doctor if they are alarming or if they continue. Here are more side effects:

- Dizziness, feeling faint, lightheadedness, especially when rising from a lying or sitting position
- Muscle cramps, spasms, pain, stiffness, trembling, jerking (with entacapone)
- Pain, burning, or discomfort: crawling, itching, numbness, prickling, "pins and needles," "tingling"; chest pain, discomfort, tightness; headache, leg pain, stomach pain, pain in back or side, jaw, neck, arms, shoulder, knees, ankles; pain with urination

- Stomach or digestive problems: belching, indigestion, burning sensation, upper abdominal pain, constipation, diarrhea, gas
- Vision changes (blurred vision)

Finally, If you have diabetes, levodopa can distort at-home blood-sugar test results. If you are diabetic and do at-home testing, be sure to discuss the possible distortion with your doctor.

Dopamine Agonists

Drugs called *dopamine agonists* mimic the effects of dopamine in the brain and give relief from PD symptoms. Commonly prescribed dopamine agonists include *bromocriptine (Parlodel), pramipexole (Mirapex), ropinirole (Requip, Requip XL),* and *apomorphine (Apokyn injection).*

Dopamine agonists may be used alone or in combination with levodopa. They often allow a reduction in the dosage of levodopa by 5 to 30 percent. Though generally not as effective as levodopa, dopamine agonists may be particularly helpful during the early stages of PD and might even equal the effectiveness of levodopa for the first one to three years of use. Once taken, it takes about seven hours for the drug to be used up.

Dopamine agonists may:

- reduce or eliminate many side effects of levodopa, including wearing-off and on-off episodes
- reduce the dosage of levodopa needed
- calm nighttime leg cramping
- be useful at any stage of the disease
- help control tremors, rigidity, and slow movements

Potential Side Effects of Dopamine Agonists

Side effects of dopamine agonists are usually temporary, but you should report them to your doctor if they are alarming or if they continue. Dopamine agonists, for example, can stimulate the pleasure center and contribute to compulsive behaviors, such as shopping, gambling, or hypersexuality. Your doctor might want to reduce the dosage or discontinue the drug if any of the following occur:

- Abnormal dreams
- Agitation
- Behavioral changes, such as uncontrollable gambling
- Unusual or uncontrolled body movements
- Drowsiness, falling asleep without warning
- Nightmares
- Sexual side effects (increased libido, hypersexuality; painful or prolonged penile erection; or loss of sex drive and ability)
- Excessive sweating

Since the drug *apomorphine* is injected, you might experience bleeding, blistering, burning, coldness, skin discoloration (redness), a feeling of pressure, infection, inflammation, itching, lumps, numbness, pain, rash (including hives), scarring, pain (soreness, stinging, or tenderness), swelling, tingling, ulceration, or warmth at the injection site. Notify your doctor as soon as possible if these symptoms occur. If they are particularly severe or alarming, follow your doctor's instructions for what to do in case of emergency.

Anticholinergics

For many years, *anticholinergics* were the primary drugs used to treat PD. These drugs reduce tremors by blocking the action of a brain chemical called *acetylcho-line*. Anticholinergics may also help prevent excessive sweating and drooling. Commonly prescribed anticholinergics are *trihexyphenidyl HCI (Artane), biperiden (Akineton), benztropine mesylate (Cogentin),* and *procyclidine (Kemadrin).*

It's estimated that anticholinergics help about half of those for whom they are prescribed. Some patients respond for a short time, and most report about 30 percent improvement. The drugs may be prescribed for mild to moderate symptoms but are usually not effective in later stages of PD. The therapeutic dosage depends on which anticholinergic is used and on the individual's response to the drug.

Potential Side Effects of Anticholinergics

Side effects are usually temporary, but you should report them to your doctor if they are alarming or if they continue. Your doctor might want to reduce the dosage or discontinue the drug if you experience any of these symptoms:

- Blurred vision
- Clumsiness, unsteadiness
- Confusion
- Dizziness or fainting (especially in a hot tub or sauna)
- Drowsiness (severe)
- Hallucinations
- Increased heart rate (more common among the elderly)
- Irritability
- Memory loss

- Nausea
- Skin changes (unusual warmth, dryness, redness)

Antiviral Medication

The antiviral medication *amantadine (Symmetrel)* is sometimes used to treat the flu. The anti-Parkinson's effects of this drug were discovered by accident when it was used to treat influenza in people who happened to have PD. The drug may be used alone or in combination with other anti-Parkinson drugs such as anticholinergics or levodopa. Amantadine has been found to decrease involuntary movements (dyskinesia)—improving muscle control and reducing stiffness and shakiness—in some PD patients. Scientists theorize that amantadine works by stimulating dopamine receptors in the brain.

Potential Side Effects of Amantadine

Side effects are usually temporary, but you should report them to your doctor if they are alarming or if they continue. Your doctor might want to reduce the dosage or discontinue the drug if any of the following occur:

- Blurred vision
- Constipation or diarrhea
- Hallucinations
- Memory loss
- Mood changes (depression, thoughts of suicide, attempts at suicide, agitation, anxiety, nervousness, irritability)
- Nightmares, other sleeping problems.
- If this drug stops working, it might start working again after being discontinued for a while.

Enzyme Inhibitors

Enzymes are molecules that increase the rates of chemical reactions, which convert one substance into another. You probably encounter enzyme-containing products every day—in laundry products that act on blood or fat stains, or in meat tenderizers that break down proteins. *Enzyme inhibitors* slow or block enzyme activity. In treating Parkinson's disease symptoms, enzyme inhibitors keep your PD drugs from "breaking down" before they reach the brain, or from breaking down too fast once they reach the brain.

There are two major types of enzyme inhibitors: *monoamine oxidase type B (MAO-B) inhibitors* and *catechol-O-methyltransferase (COMT)* inhibitors.

MAO-B Inhibitors

Monoamine oxidase type B (MAO-B) inhibitors work by blocking the *MAO-B enzyme*, which "breaks down" dopamine within the brain. The goal is to keep dopamine at its brain receptors as long as possible before being broken down by MAO-B. The MAO-B inhibitors prescribed for Parkinson's disease are *selegiline (Eldepryl, Deprenyl), selegiline hydrochloride (Zydis selegiline),* and *rasagiline (Azilect).*

Selegiline

Selegiline, which is sold as *Eldepryl* and *Deprenyl,* may be used during any stage of PD. Taken early in the disease, selegiline may reduce symptoms and delay the need to take levodopa for several months. The drug may also be used with levodopa to smooth out motor functions and to prolong "on" time.

Some researchers theorize that selegiline may actually slow the progression of PD by protecting neurons in the brain; however, this has not been proven. Evidence-based guidelines issued by the American Academy of Neurology (ANA) and the Movement Disorder Society (MDS) conclude that there is insufficient evidence to show that the drug works to protect the brain of PD patients.

Rasagiline

Like selegiline, *rasagiline*, sold as *Azilect*, prevents the enzyme MAO-B from breaking down dopamine, thus prolonging the availability of dopamine at the brain's receptors. Doctors may prescribe rasagiline early on as monotherapy, while the brain is still producing dopamine, and later in the disease to improve the effectiveness of levodopa.

Potential Side Effects of MAO-B Inhibitors

The possible side effects of these drugs include nausea, insomnia, hallucinations or confusion, and *orthostatic hypotension*, which is dizziness caused by a drop in blood pressure when you rise from a chair or bed. People taking certain antidepressants may not be good candidates for MAO-B inhibitors; the combination of the drugs may cause high blood pressure. Patients are also asked to avoid certain types of cheese, fermented meats, and fermented soy products. The amino acid *tyramine* in these foods can cause adverse reactions.

COMT Inhibitors

Catechol-O-methyl transferase (COMT) is an enzyme that breaks down levodopa before it reaches the brain. Used in combination with levodopa, COMT inhibitors prevent this chemical action, "protecting" levodopa until it gets inside the brain, where it is converted into dopamine. The

COMT inhibitors prescribed for Parkinson's disease are *entacapone (Comtan)* and *tolcapone (Tasmar)*.

Entacapone

Sold as Comtan, entacapone, is believed to be the safer of the COMT inhibitors and is more commonly prescribed than tolcapone. As mentioned earlier, the combination drug Stalevo contains entacapone along with levodopa and carbidopa.

Tolcapone

Your doctor may prescribe tolcapone, sold by the brand name Tasmar, in combination with Sinemet, making the transition from "on and off" periods smoother. It may take several months to realize the full benefit of tolcapone. Therapy with tolcapone may:

- result in a smooth response to Sinemet.
- decrease "wearing-off" periods.
- prolong the action of dopamine.
- allow up to a 25 percent reduction in the dosage of levodopa.
- prolong blood and brain levels of levodopa.
- reduce levels of potentially damaging free radicals.
- allow a reduction in the dosage of dopamine agonists in combination therapy.
- improve balance and motor activities.
- act as a stimulant and reduce feelings of fatigue.

In rare cases, tolcapone has caused serious (sometimes fatal) liver problems. Therefore, this medication should be used only in carefully selected patients. Tell your doctor if you have liver problems or difficulty controlling body movements (dyskinesia or dystonia) before you use this medication. Your doctor will test your liver function before, during, and after treatment with this medication.

If you do not notice any benefit within three weeks of starting talcopone, this medication must be stopped because liver problems could occur. Stop using this drug and notify your doctor immediately if you develop any of the following signs of liver problems: yellowing of the eyes or skin, unusual fatigue, loss of appetite, dark urine, nausea, or abdominal/stomach pain.

Potential Side Effects of COMT Inhibitors

Side effects are usually temporary, but you should report them to your doctor if they are alarming or if they continue. Your doctor may reduce the dosage or discontinue the drug if any of the following occur:

- Signs of liver damage, such as dark urine; light-colored stools; chronic nausea; loss of appetite; abdominal tenderness; feeling especially drowsy, sluggish, tired, or weak; yellow eyes or skin
- Agitation
- Behavioral or mood changes (irritability)
- Chest pain
- Confusion
- Dizziness or lightheadedness when getting up from a lying or sitting position
- Drowsiness
- Fever or chills
- Hyperactivity
- Muscle cramps, spasms, pain, stiffness, trembling, jerking
- Sore throat

- Twitching, twisting, or other unusual body movements
- Urinary problems (bloody, cloudy, or brighter yellow or orange urine; difficult, frequent, or painful urination)

Rivastigmine

Rivastigmine, whose brand name is *Exelon,* is a *cholinesterase inhibitor* used to treat a person who has both Alzheimer's disease and Parkinson's disease. The brain chemical *acetylcholine* (ACh) helps the brain work better; Parkinson's disease reduces the brain's supply of this chemical. Rivastigmine slows the breakdown of acetylcholine, helping PD patients think more clearly.

The side effects of Rivastigmine are usually temporary, but you should report them to your doctor if they are alarming or if they continue. Seizures and signs of shock (enlarged pupils; irregular breathing; fast, weak pulse) are medical emergencies. Other potential side effects include any of the following:

- Diarrhea or constipation
- Dizziness, fainting
- Excessive saliva (mouth watering)
- Excessive sweating
- Fatigue
- Hallucinations
- Nausea, vomiting
- Stomach pain or cramping
- Trouble sleeping

Using Medications Safely

Throughout this chapter, we've discussed potential side effects of medications. If you're having any side effects or adverse reactions to a drug, call your doctor or go to an emergency room immediately. Make sure you understand the possible side effects and drug interactions each time you begin using a new drug. Ask your doctor whether you should wear a Medic-Alert bracelet.

On rare occasions, PD patients experience dangerous drug-allergy reactions such as:

- Hives, itching, rash
- Swelling of the face, lips, tongue, and/or throat
- Difficulty in breathing or swallowing

An allergic reaction is a medical emergency. Call 9-1-1, have someone take you to a nearby hospital emergency room, or follow your doctor's instructions for what to do in case of an emergency. It is always better to be safe than sorry.

Managing Multiple Medications

To treat the symptoms of PD, you may need to take a number of medications. In many cases, you must take precisely the right dose at precisely the right time. With so many medications to keep track of, you'll want to develop an easy-to-use system that simplifies drug taking. Here are some suggestions:

Use a medication chart. Ask your doctor or pharmacist for a medication chart to keep track of your prescription and over-the-counter medications. Or make your own chart.

Keep medicines in their original containers. In general, you should keep all your drugs in their original containers to prevent dangerous mix-ups. However, if you choose to use a pill organizer, make sure that you are able to identify each medication.

Keep extra doses with you. Pack a few doses of medication, a can of juice, and some crackers in your car, office, and places you visit frequently. Or keep a fanny pack loaded with your prescriptions and juice.

Remind yourself when to take your medications. There are a number of ways to do this. Set your watch or alarm clock. Put the drugs where you will see them. For instance, if you take medicine first thing in the morning, put it in the bathroom by your toothbrush or in the kitchen where you eat breakfast. Be sure to always keep your medications out of the reach of children.

Have one doctor oversee your medications. If you have several health problems and more than one doctor, you are at higher risk for dangerous drug interactions. Ask your primary health care provider or your neurologist to oversee *all* your medications.

Keep a list of all your drugs and dosages. Take that list with you to the hospital, emergency room, dentist's office, and doctor's office. All medical professionals you are working with should know exactly what drugs you're taking.

Choose one pharmacy. Find a pharmacist who will keep track of all your drugs and alert you of potentially dangerous drug interactions. Most pharmacies are now computerized, which makes drug tracking much easier.

Don't change your dosage or stop taking medications without first talking to your doctor. Your physician may recommend that you gradually taper off these drugs to reduce the chance of side effects.

Never use someone else's drugs. You can never be sure it is the exact same drug you're used to taking.

Never use old or outdated drugs. They may have lost their potency.

Use a pill cutter. If your prescription requires that you take half a pill, pill cutters are available at pharmacies. To keep pills from crumbling when you cut them, place them in a freezer for an hour beforehand. If you have trouble cutting the pills, ask someone else to do it. Do not cut extended-release or slow-release pills.

A Word about Taking Drugs for Life

You might be uncomfortable with the idea of taking drugs for the rest of your life. Some people are opposed to drug therapy and try to treat PD the "natural way," with various diet regimens, herbs and concoctions from health-food stores, and vitamin and mineral supplements. However, no current evidence suggests that you can control PD symptoms "naturally," without chemical replacement therapy, any more than you can control diabetes without insulin.

At least for now, effectively treating PD means taking medications. Many of these medications can bring you relief from symptoms, but you need to be patient. Naturally, you want relief from your symptoms as quickly as possible. However, with many PD drugs you might not notice any effect for several days, weeks, or even months. When your doctor prescribes a new drug, you'll probably start with a low dose that will be gradually increased to make sure that the drug is safe for you.

6

Surgery as Treatment for Parkinson's Disease

Neurosurgery to treat PD symptoms was first performed in the 1930s and was fairly common until the 1960s and the development of l-dopa. Surgery is still an option for those who can't take l-dopa or other anti-Parkinson drugs, or who have severe motor symptoms—rigidity, bradykinesia (slowness of movement), akinesia (absence of movement), or tremor—despite drug treatment.

The four types of surgical procedures for PD are: deep-brain stimulation, pallidotomy, thalamotomy, and neural implants. These procedures are described in the text that follows.

Deep-Brain Stimulation (DBS)

PD symptoms are triggered by abnormal electrical nerve signals from the brain. High-tech imaging techniques such as *computed tomography* (CT) scanning, *magnetic resonance imaging* (MRI), and *microelectric recording* can find the precise area of the brain where the abnormal signals originate.

In *deep-brain stimulation* surgery, a neurosurgeon implants an electrode into that area of the brain—either the

Deep-Brain Stimulation

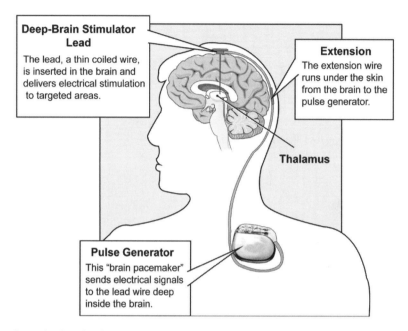

Deep-Brain Stimulator Lead
The lead, a thin coiled wire, is inserted in the brain and delivers electrical stimulation to targeted areas.

Extension
The extension wire runs under the skin from the brain to the pulse generator.

Thalamus

Pulse Generator
This "brain pacemaker" sends electrical signals to the lead wire deep inside the brain.

Deep-brain stimulation reduces Parkinson's symptoms related to movement—tremors, slowness, stiffness, and gait problems.

subthalamic nucleus (STN) or the internal *globus pallidus (GPi)*. A wire beneath the skin connects the electrode to a battery-operated neurostimulator (similar to a heart pacemaker) implanted in your chest. The neurostimulator, which is programmed by your surgeon, sends pulses to the electrode that block the abnormal nerve signals and thus relieve PD symptoms. You will receive a controller so you can turn the device on and off and make certain adjustments, if necessary.

The response to surgery will be only as good as the best response to levodopa. DBS can be used in the following brain locations: *thalamus (Vim), subthalamic nucleus (STN),* and *globus pallidus (GPi).*

Deep-brain stimulation is painless (amazingly, the brain itself is insensitive to pain) and is the most common surgical procedure for treating PD symptoms. It is actually two operations performed consecutively—one to implant the electrode in the brain, and the second to implant the neurostimulator and battery pack in your chest. It is necessary for you to be awake and to communicate with the surgeon during the first operation.

The battery will last several years—the newest models up to ten years—before a new one must be inserted via a minor surgical procedure. And, unlike other forms of brain surgery for PD, deep-brain stimulation is reversible.

Potential Complications and Side Effects of Deep-Brain Stimulation

You might need several follow-up visits with your surgeon to fine-tune the neurostimulator settings and get rid of side effects such as worsening of symptoms, tingling sensations, and numbness.

In addition to the brain-surgery risks already mentioned, there are rare complications of deep-brain stimulation, including electrode breakage or infection and visual flashes (from improper electrode placement).

Are You a Good Candidate for Deep-Brain Stimulation?

Deep-brain stimulation is not effective for everyone. Patients who received little or no relief from levodopa/carbidopa will likely not benefit from this surgery. You might be a good candidate for deep-brain stimulation if you have benefited from levodopa/carbidopa therapy and these drugs are losing their effectiveness. You need to be physically and mentally able to undergo the operation.

Pallidotomy

First introduced in the 1940s, *pallidotomy* involves inserting a probe in the brain and destroying a part of the brain tissue called the *globus pallidus*, which is involved in the transmission of brain signals for movement. A successful pallidotomy can improve gait and reduce or eliminate tremors, slowness of movement, abnormal movements, stiffness, balance difficulties, and freezing. PD patients who do well following a pallidotomy take less l-dopa or are able to take it with better results.

During pallidotomy, a halo frame is placed over the head of the patient. A picture of the brain is taken by MRI or CT scan. Under local anesthesia the patient is able to describe sensations as the surgery progresses. A larger metal frame, or *stereotactic frame*, is placed over the halo frame to guide the insertion of a probe deep into the globus pallidus, and the surgeon drills a small hole in the skull. Once the probe is in the proper position, the doctor applies an electrical current through the probe into the pallidum, lesioning it. If the surgery works well, the patient's abnormal movements disappear immediately. Often, the tremors as well as the slowness and rigidity subside.

Some surgeons believe that the globus pallidus should be lesioned on both sides of the brain for best results. Others contend the procedure should be performed only on one side. It's clear that bilateral procedures carry greater risk. At this time, most authorities do not recommend the two-sided procedure.

Although both pallidotomy and thalamotomy (described below) have been made safer and more effective with the use of imaging techniques such as MRI and CT scans and frames, the procedures still carry risks of potentially serious complications. Some of the side effects following surgery, however, are only temporary.

Potential Complications of Pallidotomy

- Stroke caused by bleeding from damaged blood vessels
- Confusion
- Sleepiness
- Weakness of facial muscles
- Weakness of arm and leg muscles
- Speech difficulties
- Problems swallowing
- Personality changes
- Problems concentrating
- Increase in appetite and weight gain
- Visual problems, including partial vision loss or (rarely) blindness
- Balance problems when walking

Are You a Good Candidate for Pallidotomy?

You may be a candidate for pallidotomy if you

- are severely disabled and have failed to respond to all anti-Parkinson medications.
- are unable to take anti-Parkinson medications, or if medications are ineffective or worsen symptoms.
- are younger than age seventy.
- are mentally competent.

- have a tremor, abnormal movements (dyskinesias), and motor fluctuations.

- are in good general health.

Thalamotomy

Thalamotomy destroys a small portion of the thalamus, a message-relay station deep inside the brain. When performed on one side of the brain, a thalamotomy often relieves severe tremors on the opposite side of the body. First introduced in the 1940s, thalamotomy gained favor because it reduced PD tremors more effectively than did pallidotomy. New surgical techniques have made the procedure safer; however, it is not without possible complications.

Potential Complications of Thalamotomy

- Convulsions or seizures

- Disturbances in gait and balance

- Severe speech and swallowing difficulties, especially when the thalamotomy has been performed on both sides of the thalamus

- Problems with memory

- Bleeding into the brain (mortality less than 1 percent)

Are You a Good Candidate for Thalamotomy?

About 60 percent of PD patients experience tremor. Of this group, about 10 percent suffer from disabling tremor and stand to gain the most from the surgery. This procedure may be an option for you if you are

- experiencing tremor not relieved by PD drugs.

- unable to carry out the activities of daily living.

69

- disabled occupationally or socially.

Neural Implants

In the 1980s, neurosurgeons in Sweden and China tried transplanting bits of live brain tissue from aborted fetuses into the brains of PD patients. The idea was that if these cells "took hold," they might make the brain produce more dopamine. However, success with this procedure has been slow, and moral controversy gave rise to a long-standing ban on fetal-tissue research. The ban was lifted in 1993, making further exploration of this surgery possible. Still, there are still plenty of unanswered questions, and the surgery is considered experimental. It will likely be ten or more years before neural implants produce any real hope for treatment.

If you are considering surgery to relieve your PD symptoms, choose your surgeon carefully. He or she should be a board-certified neurosurgeon who is experienced in the procedure and who is a Fellow in the American College of Surgeons.

7

The Importance of Exercise

Regular exercise is one of the most important self-help strategies for coping with PD. The phrase "use it or lose it" definitely applies when it comes to PD. That's not to say it's easy. Nearly everyone has difficulty staying fit. Most avoid exercise altogether or try a few sessions and quit. If you have PD, exercise might be especially unappealing due to fatigue, limited movement, stiffness in the muscles and joints, or breathing problems.

Research and the experiences of thousands of people with PD confirm that exercise is vitally important for motor function. A study at Emory University School of Medicine in Atlanta, Georgia, found that both stretching exercise and aerobic exercise are helpful for those with PD. Study participants walked or ran forty minutes per day three times a week for twelve weeks. At the end of the trial, their cardiovascular fitness improved by more than 30 percent, their motor function improved by 22 percent, and their movement time improved by 37 percent.

Exercise will not stop PD, but it may give you greater strength and independence. It may also improve balance, help you overcome gait problems, strengthen particular muscles, and improve speech and swallowing. If you exercise vigorously enough to work up at least a light sweat, you may feel better emotionally and improve symptoms of depression, because exercise releases endorphins, the body's own "feel-good" chemicals. Perhaps most important, a regular exercise program may help you feel more in control and give you a sense of accomplishment. A structured exercise class or program that allows you to regularly connect with others will help you feel less isolated.

Research shows that exercise helps prevent muscle and joint injury commonly associated with PD. Each day you perform thousands of automatic movements with your body, continuously stretching your ligaments and muscles. When PD interferes with automatic movement, you must consciously think out each movement before performing it; your muscles and ligaments may stiffen and your joints lose their range of motion. If you try to perform movements that are beyond the limited range or capacity of the ligaments and muscles, injuries such as sprains or strains are likely. Exercise can delay this process and protect your muscles and ligaments from damage.

Benefits of Exercise

A regular exercise program may help you:

- increase muscle strength.
- improve balance.
- overcome gait problems.
- decrease speech/swallowing problems.
- improve mood and lift depression.
- reduce muscle and joint injuries.
- feel more in control.
- gain a sense of accomplishment.
- feel more connected and less isolated.

Exercise that Works for You

Many PD patients give high priority to regular aerobic, stretching, and strengthening exercises in their treatment plans. Below are suggestions for safe and effective exercise. (Check with your doctor before you start *any* exercise regimen.)

Begin slowly. Muscles and joints unaccustomed to physical activity respond slowly. Start slowly and increase activity gradually over time. Trying to do too much too soon will only result in sore muscles and possible injury.

Choose an exercise regimen that you can easily fit into your daily routine. Your exercise plan should be one that you can and will do consistently and that you enjoy, which will motivate you to stick with it.

If it hurts, stop. Don't push yourself to the point of pain. Slight discomfort is okay, but pain is a definite signal from your body to stop. If exercise consistently causes pain, talk with your doctor, your physical therapist, or both.

Practice proper walking. Take large steps, lifting your toes when you begin a step and letting your heels hit the floor first as you step forward. Practice walking sideways, backward, and in circles several times a day.

Lift your toes. To prevent stumbling, raise your toes from the walking surface with every step. Also use toe lifting to "unglue" your feet and legs from a freezing episode, to relieve muscle spasms, and to reduce the possibility of a fall.

Create a wide base. When standing, walking, or turning, keep your feet about twelve inches apart to provide a wider base and help prevent falling.

Turn with small steps. Practice turning with a wide stance and small steps for at least fifteen minutes every day until it becomes habitual.

Look up. When walking, you might be tempted to watch your feet. Try to straighten up and look straight ahead.

Practice rapid movements. To improve your balance, move rapidly forward, backward, to the right, and to the left for five minutes at a time several times a day.

Overcome gravity. If getting out of a chair or bed is a problem, practice rising very quickly to overcome inertia and the pull of gravity. Be sure both feet are planted firmly beneath your chair or bed. Practice ten to twenty times a day. Put three- or four-inch safely blocks under the back legs of your favorite chair to make getting up easier. Some chairs are mechanized to "propel" you forward and out of the chair. Don't invest in one before asking your neurologist whether such chairs are safe for you.

Swing your arms. When you walk, practice swinging your arms freely—taking pressure off your legs, lessening fatigue, and loosening the arms and shoulders. As one arm swings forward, the other should swing back. As your right arm moves forward, swing your left leg forward, and vice versa.

Balance the list. Some people with PD find themselves listing to one side or another. Try carrying hand weights or a shopping bag loaded with books on the nonlisting side to balance the load and decrease your body's bend.

Consider an in-home exercise machine. Bad weather can make it easy to put off exercising. Treadmills, stationary bikes, and other in-home exercise machines will help you stick to your regimen.

March to the music. Try using music to help you maintain a steady gait, especially if you're experiencing freezing problems. Music can also make your exercise more interesting and enjoyable.

Keep your legs strong. Be sure to include some exercises that improve your leg strength. Strong legs will enable you to remain active longer and can prevent falls.

Strengthen those abs. Strong stomach muscles are important, especially if you suffer from back pain. Make sure your exercise routine includes "crunches," modified sit-ups, or other abdomen-strengthening exercises recommended or approved by your doctor.

Try yoga. This ancient art has a number of gentle stretching and strengthening postures that you should find quite helpful with posture, balance, relaxation, and serenity. Even people who are bedridden can use some of the postures. Talk to the instructor before you sign up for a yoga class, however, because some forms of yoga are physically demanding.

Avoid rubber- or crepe-soled shoes. They can grip the floor and trip you.

Practice, practice, practice. If any task proves difficult, such as buttoning a shirt or getting out of bed, practice it at least twenty times a day to improve performance.

A Word about Expectations

Your expectations should be realistic. Before you had PD, you may have worked out and quickly made noticeable gains in muscle strength and cardiovascular endurance. It will be different with PD.

Don't be discouraged if your muscle strength and endurance show little or no improvement. Your disease is continuing to progress. Your exercise program is simply helping you keep pace with the progression of symptoms, especially the more disabling ones. If the exercise is helping you maintain a better quality of life and giving you a sense of control and accomplishment, then be proud of your achievements.

What Kind of Exercise Should You Do?

All kinds of exercises may help. Your choice depends on your symptoms, your age, your physical strength, and your interests. The best program is one that combines a number of activities and continually changes as your symptoms and capabilities change. Your doctor and your physical therapist can help you develop a program that is right for you.

Daily-activities exercise. This is the work you do as part of day-to-day living—household chores, bathing, dressing, grooming, shopping, and so on. Although this type of exercise won't improve your aerobic endurance (heart and lung fitness), it will help you stay limber.

Doctor-prescribed activities. Your doctor may prescribe special exercises to prevent muscle stiffness and worsening of other symptoms, or to recover functions that you may have lost.

Other preventive exercises. Preventive walking exercises are especially helpful. For instance, walking with a deliberately wide gait and small steps—your eyes focused straight ahead—is a good exercise to straighten your posture, improve gait, and prevent falling.

Corrective exercises. Repetitively practice these exercises to overcome movement limitations at particular joints. Getting out of a chair rapidly over and over will improve mobility of your hip and leg joints.

Recreational exercises. Participate as much as you can in fun activities such as golfing, dancing, bowling, swimming, hiking, and other forms of exercise you enjoy. Recreation can help your muscles and joints remain flexible and strong, and also provides social opportunities.

A Sample Exercise Routine

A good exercise program combines stretching exercises (to keep joints and muscles limber) with strengthening exercises. Many of the exercises suggested below are adaptations of yoga postures. Some or all of these exercises may work well for you, but check first with your doctor, your physical therapist, or both. The entire regimen should take about an hour.

Walking. For at least thirty minutes, walk as vigorously as possible outdoors or on a treadmill. Your physical therapist can recommend a good walking shoe.

Proper breathing. During exercise, exhale while you're doing the "work" part of an exercise—stretching or lifting a weight, for example. Inhale as you do the relaxation part of the exercise. Breathing this way will prevent injuries and make the exercises easier.

Low back stretch. Lie flat on your back and bend your knees. Clasp your knees with your hands, pulling your legs toward your chest. You will feel a stretch in your lower back. Hold for a slow count of ten. Repeat this exercise as often as you like. It's a great way to loosen a stiff back in the morning.

Long body stretch. Lying flat on your back, raise your arms over your head and stretch your entire body as far as you can.

Shoulder stretch. While standing, place both arms behind your back, clasping your fingers together. Straighten your arms and raise them as high as you are able. Hold the position for a count of ten—longer if you can. This is a great exercise for straightening your back.

Hip twist. Lie on the floor on your back. Bring your knees up into a slightly bent position. Now place one leg over the top of the opposite knee, allowing the upper leg to press down on the bottom leg. Keep your shoulders pressed to the floor. Let the bottom leg stretch only as far as it will comfortably go. You will feel a stretch in your lower back. Hold for a count of 20. Slowly bring your legs back to the floor. Repeat with the opposite leg.

Neck stretch. Lie on your back on the floor. Without using a pillow, rotate your head slowly back and forth from side to side. Do 15 to 20 rotations. Then raise your head, alternately tilting your neck back and pulling your chin to your chest. Repeat 25 to 50 times. These exercises will increase the range of motion in your neck and reduce stiffness.

Single-leg strap stretch. Sitting on the floor with both legs extended straight in front of you, loop a strap or towel over one foot and bend the opposite knee out to the side. Using both hands to hold the strap, pull toward your body. You should feel stretching in your lower back and the back of your leg. Hold for a count of 15 to 20. Repeat on the opposite side.

Double-leg strap stretch. Sitting on the floor with both legs extended straight in front of you, loop a strap or towel over both feet. Grasping the strap or towel with both hands, pull toward your body, stretching and holding for a count of 15 to 20.

Side stretch. Stand with a wide stance. Lift your left arm over your head, palm facing toward the midline of the body. Slowly bend your waist toward the right, allowing the weight of your raised arm to help you stretch. You should feel a stretch on your left side. Hold for a slow count of 10. Repeat on the opposite side.

Waist twist. Standing with a wide stance and with your hands on your hips, slowly twist your head and torso toward the right as far as you can. Hold for a count of 10.

Then twist back to the center and repeat on the opposite side.

Wall squats. Face the wall and stand about eight inches from it. Bend your legs at the hips and knees, lowering yourself into a squatting position. Use the wall for support if needed. Hold this position for a slow count of 10. Then slowly rise to a standing position. This exercise is excellent for leg strength, though it might be too hard for some.

Arm weight lifts. Lie on your back with a hand weight (dumbbell) no heavier than eight pounds in each hand. (Sporting-goods and discount stores usually have a good selection of hand weights as light as two pounds. Start out with smaller weights until you build up some upper-body strength.) Hold the weights parallel to your body with your elbows at your sides and your palms up. Keeping your arms straight, raise them until they are extended straight up. Hold briefly in the fully extended position, then slowly lower the weights to the starting position. Gradually work up to 50 lifts. Then begin the exercise with your arms extended from your shoulders at right angles to your body, palms facing upward, lifting them until they meet. Hold briefly and lower. Again, gradually work up to 50 lifts.

Foot-grasp back stretch. Sit on the floor with your legs extended in front of you, knees bent at about forty-five degrees. Bend your upper body forward as far as you can, extend your arms forward, and grasp the soles of your shoes with both hands. Using your back muscles, stretch toward your feet, gently lengthening your lower back. Hold for a count of 10 if possible. (Stop immediately if you feel pain.) Slowly work up to holding for at least a count of 30. This is excellent for relieving lower back pain and taking the kinks out.

Partial sit-ups with weights. Lie flat on your back. With your knees bent and your arms at your sides, grasp a hand weight in each hand. Slowly raise your upper body off the floor and curl toward your knees, keeping the small of your back and your feet on the floor. Slowly curl back down to the resting position. Gradually work up to fifty sit-ups. This exercise strengthens abdominal muscles, important for preventing lower back pain.

Physical Therapy

PD may cause problems in posture, deformities of the legs and arms, and gait disturbances. A program of physical therapy tailored to the individual may help control these problems. You, your doctor, and your physical therapist should work together to develop a program that may include:

Active and passive exercises. Active exercises are movements that can help you improve your range of motion, coordination, and speed of movement. Passive exercises include various stretches and manipulation by a physical therapist to help relieve muscle rigidity and stiffness.

Gait training. This training may improve how you walk by helping you learn proper foot placement, arm swing, and balance.

Daily-life activities. A physical therapist can help you develop techniques to make daily activities easier to accomplish.

Heat, ice, electrical stimulation, and hydrotherapy. Your physical therapist may use heat, cold, electricity, or water therapy to treat your symptoms.

Other Therapies

It is important to maintain as much coordination and manual dexterity as possible. *Occupational therapies*, including craft projects, can help. Look for activities that you enjoy and that are safe for your condition. If you develop speech difficulties, speech therapy can often help.

Speech therapists can provide exercises and techniques to overcome problems such as nasal monotone and softness in the voice.

8

Day-to-Day Coping

Coping with Parkinson's disease is challenging; it affects your entire life, from socializing with friends to earning a living. Everyday movements that used to be easy, such as buttoning your shirt or rising from a chair, can become taxing.

PD requires that you learn a new way of living, especially if you wish to remain as active as possible. This chapter offers practical coping strategies and tools for getting the assistance you need to meet the challenges of daily life.

Finding Support

Finding emotional support is important if you're living with PD. Many organizations—such as the National Parkinson Foundation and the Parkinson's Disease Foundation (see Resources at the back of this book)—sponsor support groups for people with PD and their loved ones. These support groups include patients, patient/partner, caregiver, young-onset PD patients, as well as groups for the entire family.

Many people, especially those newly diagnosed with PD, resist joining support groups. They prize their independence and don't want to be associated with "sick people." This initial resistance usually fades as patients come to grips with their disease.

A support group can be a vital link in your self-help education network. It may help you and your loved ones

- understand more about PD and the physical limitations imposed by the disease.

- become aware of community resources such as exercise programs, home health care services, and sources of adaptive equipment.

- obtain referrals to qualified health care professionals in your area who have experience with PD.

- talk about your fears and concerns in a supportive environment.

- develop ways to deal with such feelings as anger, guilt, and helplessness.

- stay motivated to use exercise and other self-help strategies.

- communicate more effectively with your health care team.

- learn about the latest developments in PD research and treatment.

- find practical ways of meeting everyday challenges.

How can you find support groups? Start with your community's local chapter of the National Parkinson Foundation or the Parkinson's Disease Foundation. If your community doesn't have a local chapter, call or write to the foundation's national headquarters (see Resources) and ask about forming a support group. You may also locate support groups through the following:

- Your local hospital
- Your doctor

- Friends or associates who have PD or a similar neurological disorder
- Your community's mental-health association
- A PD research center in your area

Choosing a Nutritious Diet

Eating a well-balanced diet is important for everyone's good health but especially for people with a chronic disease such as PD. No diet or nutritional supplement can cure PD or slow the progression of the disease. Even so, diet is important both for your overall well-being and for specific aspects of your treatment. Careful food planning in consultation with a dietitian may prevent many diet-related problems.

Here are just some of the dietary issues involved in Parkinson's disease:

- Swallowing may be difficult or slow.

- PD slows the rate at which food moves through the digestive tract. It takes longer for the stomach to empty. With the slowing of digestion, constipation may become a problem.

- Some people with PD experience decreased appetite, changes in smell, and nausea (from anti-Parkinson medications), all of which may make eating less enjoyable and cause weight loss.

- A poor diet (or one that's high in protein) may interfere with the absorption of anti-Parkinson drugs such as levodopa.

Generally speaking, people with PD require the same nutrients as those recommended for everyone. Many of the same standards of good eating apply. A few additional dietary principles are especially helpful for people with PD.

Variety. Eat a variety of foods every day. Include vege-tables, fruits, whole-grain breads, pasta, rice, legumes, eggs, meat, poultry, and fish.

Fat. Stick to a low-fat diet. High-fat diets have been linked to heart disease. Be especially wary of foods loaded with saturated fat and cholesterol, such as fatty red meats. Decrease the amount of fat in your diet by eating lean meat, fish, and skinless poultry and cutting down on butter, oil, cheese, and ice cream. Drink low-fat milk. Substitute other lower-fat dairy products for higher-fat ones. If you need to add calories to your diet, complex carbohydrates are a better source than fats.

Complex carbohydrates. Carbohydrates that come from whole grains (in bread, rolls, and pasta, for example) are usually better choices than simple carbohydrates such as sugar and baked goods made with white flour. Complex carbohydrates are good sources of energy-rich nutrients and of fiber (necessary for regular bowel movements).

Fiber. Fiber, the indigestible parts of plants, may pre-vent constipation. You may get fiber in your diet from whole grains, fruits, and vegetables.

Water. Drink plenty of water throughout the day. It aids in many body processes, including digestion, nutrient absorption, blood circulation, and excretion of toxins and waste. Furthermore, water helps your body absorb medica-tions and, of course, prevents dehydration.

Most experts recommend drinking six to eight 8-ounce glasses of water every day. Don't wait until you're thirsty. Our sense of thirst diminishes with age, and anti-Parkinson drugs may have a drying effect. Drinking plain water—not coffee, tea, cola, or other drinks containing caffeine or sugar—is the best way to stay hydrated.

Weight. Weigh yourself weekly. If you're overweight, you'll find it harder to move around. If you weigh too little, you might not be getting enough essential nutrients (talk with your doctor or dietician about delicious liquid supplements such as Ensure or Boost). A healthy weight range and BMI (body mass index) is important for balance, mobility, and energy, so work with your dietician to reach and maintain a goal weight ideal for you.

Small, frequent meals. Because your digestion is slowed with PD, eating smaller meals throughout the day, known as "grazing," will help your body better digest and utilize foods.

Multivitamins. Some people get all the nourishment they need from a well-balanced and carefully planned diet. In the case of chronic illnesses such as PD, however, it's a good idea to take a multivitamin-mineral supplement as "nutritional insurance."

Ask your doctor to recommend a nutritional supplement that contains a good supply of *antioxidants* to fight *free-radical* damage. Free radicals are unstable molecules that "seek out" and then bind with other particles in the body. Excess free radicals can harm normal cells. Emotional stress, smoking, and poor nutrition are known causes of excess free radicals.

Antioxidants, such as vitamins C and E and selenium, can bond with and neutralize free radicals. The role of antioxidants in treating PD symptoms is unclear. Scientists have theorized that vitamins C and E may slow the progression of PD, but research has yet to confirm this hypothesis.

In any case, it's a good idea to take nutritional supplements, including antioxidants, as protection from other illnesses—especially if PD makes it harder to eat and to digest your food properly. If you currently take a nutritional supplement, show the ingredient list to your doctor or pharmacist to make sure it contains enough *but not too much* antioxidant and other nutritional benefits and that it is compatible with your medications.

Calcium. PD often strikes people over fifty, those most at risk for bone-thinning osteoporosis and related bone fractures. If you restrict your protein intake by cutting down on dairy products to improve the absorption of certain anti-Parkinson drugs, you may not be getting all the calcium you need. Be sure to get 1,000 to 1,500 milligrams of calcium each day.

Some doctors recommend *calcium citrate* combined with magnesium and vitamin D as the most beneficial form of calcium supplementation, since it contains not only the mineral itself but also the substances that enable the body to use it. Calcium supplementation is available in many forms, so ask your doctor for recommendations.

Nausea. Both PD and the medications used to treat the disease can cause nausea. Walking helps with nausea, probably because it helps food move through the digestive tract. Eating smaller meals and sipping ginger ale or ginger tea may help. (To make ginger tea, steep several peeled pieces of fresh gingerroot in hot water for an hour, then strain and serve.) Drinking a glass of juice or eating a bowl of cereal with a nonprotein, nondairy creamer is also helpful.

Digestion. During a meal, sit down, eat slowly, and chew thoroughly. Avoid eating on the run. It's bad for digestion and may cause you to inhale food into your airways.

Overcoming Sleep Problems

Getting a good night's sleep can be a problem for anyone. Sleep difficulties increase gradually after age thirty-five and are especially bothersome for people with PD. Chronic sleep problems leave you feeling fatigued and can aggravate PD symptoms. Common PD-related sleep difficulties include the problems listed below:

- Waking several times during the night
- Waking early in the morning and being unable to get back to sleep
- Having nightmares
- Being sleepy during the day

Some PD-related sleep problems are caused by changes in the brain and nervous system and the muscles. For instance, researchers have found that levels of the brain chemical *serotonin*, important for deep sleep, are lower in people with PD. Difficulty falling asleep may be related to depression, persistent tremors, nighttime leg cramping, restless-leg syndrome, or rigidity and the inability to turn over. Early-morning awakening may occur as medications wear off or result from depression and anxiety. Nightmares, vivid dreaming, thrashing, and walking or talking in your sleep might be side effects of levodopa. Some people with PD have trouble sleeping at night because they nap during the day.

Sleep disturbances may pose problems not only for you but also for your partner or caregiver. Interrupted sleep may leave you both exhausted, lacking the reserves of energy you need for effectively coping with PD. If your sleep problems are mild to moderate, the suggestions below may help you get a better night's sleep. If not, talk to your physician about effective sleep medications.

Accept that you need less sleep. As we age, our bodies require less sleep. If you're accustomed to the luxury of "sleeping in," you may have difficulty adjusting to this physiological change.

Break up your sleep. Don't be afraid to divide your sleep into two periods—a short nap in the afternoon and a longer stretch at night.

Avoid oversleeping. Sleep only as much as necessary to feel refreshed when you wake. Too much sleep—a common depression symptom—may leave you feeling unrested.

Go to bed and get up at the same time every day. Sticking to a schedule helps regulate your internal clock, which, in turn, regulates your sleep–wake cycle.

Exercise regularly. Research has shown that although sporadic exercising does not improve sleep quality, regular moderate exercise deepens sleep. Make sure you finish your exercise routine at least an hour before going to bed.

Turn down the sound. Many people are light sleepers, easily distracted by noises. Wear earplugs or turn on a fan or white-noise sound machine to muffle external sounds.

Darken the room. Even small amounts of light may interrupt sleep. Try using heavy curtains or shades to block out light.

Sleep cool. Trying to sleep in a room that is too warm may disturb slumber. Turn down the furnace and crack a window for fresh air to keep your bedroom at a comfortable sleeping temperature.

Avoid caffeine. Many people have difficulty sleeping after they ingest coffee, tea, cola, chocolate, or other beverages or foods containing caffeine. If you need a warm drink before bed, try herbal tea or milk. Warm milk can be especially relaxing because it contains tryptophan, an ingredient that helps induce sleep.

Limit alcohol. A glass of wine or another alcoholic beverage helps some people fall asleep. But alcohol also tends to fragment sleep and may cause "rebound" awakenings. If you consume alcohol, do so several hours before retiring.

Avoid liquids after 6 p.m. Many people are awakened during the night by a full bladder. If this commonly happens to you, forgo the warm-milk remedy and other drinks in the evening. Also, be sure to urinate right before going to bed.

Eat a snack. Hunger may interfere with sleep. Try crackers and cheese, a piece of toast, or warm milk and honey to take the edge off hunger and help induce sleep. Carbohydrates may help calm you and make you sleepy.

Stop smoking. Cigarette, pipe, and cigar smoking are bad for your general health. Chronic tobacco use may also disturb sleep.

Watch what you watch. Violent TV programs or movies, cliffhangers, or emotionally disturbing videos aren't likely to put you in the mood for sleep.

Reserve your bed for sleep. Some sleep experts recommend using your bed only for sleep, not for reading, watching television, doing crossword puzzles, finishing paperwork, or performing other activities that are better done in the living room or den. That way, when you get into bed, your mind associates your bed only with sleep.

Try separate beds. If you're rested in the morning but your partner isn't, try separate beds or bedrooms. PD-related nightmares, shouting, or thrashing can disturb your partner's sleep more than your own.

Ask about adjusting your medications. If PD symptoms wake you up or if you have to be awake in order to turn over, talk with your doctor. Find out if your medications may be adjusted to better control your symptoms at night.

Go with the flow. If you can't sleep, don't fight it. Get up and read, watch TV, or do some other activity until you feel sleepy.

Try a sleep aid. After two nights of poor sleep, consider taking a sleep medication prescribed by your doctor.

Coping with Speech and Swallowing Difficulties

Experts familiar with PD estimate that 60 to 90 percent of PD patients have speech difficulties and about half have trouble swallowing. These problems may be subtle or debilitating.

Speech and swallowing are complex processes that involve many nerves and muscles of the lower face, lips, tongue, voice box, throat, and chest. Just as the automatic muscle movements involved in walking may be affected by PD, so may the automatic muscle and nerve functions involved in speaking and swallowing. In addition, speech and swallowing may be interrupted by bothersome involuntary movements of the tongue and jaw.

Speaking Problems

PD-related speech problems, called *hypokinetic dysarthria,* occur when the muscles involved in speaking and breathing become stiff and rigid, causing speech to sound weak, slow, or uncoordinated. It's important to recognize that hypokinetic dysarthria does not affect intelligence, memory, or personality.

Although PD-related speech problems are unique to each individual, there are several common complaints. Some people with PD have just one of these problems, while others have multiple speech difficulties.

- Hoarse, gravelly, or breathy voice
- Loss of volume

- Difficulty changing volume
- Monotone (Normal speech uses a variety of pitches —higher and lower sounds—for expressiveness. Someone with PD might find these pitch changes difficult or impossible, thus speaking at a single pitch, in a "monotone.")
- Fast/slow speech
- Poor pronunciation

If you have any of the speech impairments listed above, see a speech therapist immediately. The sooner your speech problems are diagnosed and treated, the better the results.

You will be evaluated by a professional speech therapist, preferably a speech-language pathologist who is certified and licensed in treating speech problems. Ask your doctor, another member of your health care team, or a nearby hospital for a referral to a qualified speech therapist. If you can't find a local referral, write or call the American Speech-Language-Hearing Association in Rockville, Maryland (see Resources at the back of this book), for a referral to a speech expert in your area.

A speech therapist will help you improve the functioning of affected muscles, prescribe exercises to delay or prevent future speech problems, and advise you about other techniques to compensate for losses in your ability to communicate. Note that not everyone achieves the same outcomes with speech therapy. Effective results depend on early treatment, motivation, age, overall health, and family support.

People with mild, subtle speech changes may expect speech therapy to help them regain normal or near-normal speech. Those with moderate speech problems usually make some gains in speech and learn other ways to make themselves understood. For people with PD who can't speak intelligibly, there are alternative ways of communicating, perhaps with a machine or voice-output computer.

Speech Exercises

If you have speech problems, in addition to the strategies offered by your therapist, consider these suggestions:

- Be aware of your voice problem and work on it every day. Use a tape recorder to make yourself aware of subtle speech changes.

- Take a deep breath before speaking so that your words come out more forcefully and clearly.

- Open your mouth to let the sound out.

- Speak in short sentences.

- Clearly enunciate syllables, as professional radio announcers do. Exaggerate every sound in every syllable.

- Exercise your voice by reading aloud, shouting, or singing.

- In front of a mirror, practice expressing emotions with your face muscles. Show anger, happiness, sorrow, surprise.

- Let your listeners know about your speech difficulty, and ask them to let you know when they can't hear or understand you.

Your speech therapist will likely give you a number of exercises, depending on your particular speech difficulties. The following exercises, recommended by national PD organizations, may help you reduce muscle rigidity and regain control of the muscles involved in speech. Do the exercises in front of a mirror daily. (Many of these exercises also help with swallowing difficulties.)

Deep breathing. Take five deep breaths, stretching out the stomach muscles as you breathe in, tightening them as you breathe out. Exhale fully, for as long as you can, before taking the next breath.

Vowel breathing. Take five deep breaths, adding vowel sounds such as "ah," "oh," and "oo" as you exhale.

Automatic speech. Practice reciting strings of words such as the days of the week, the months of the year, and the alphabet. Be sure to provide good breath support for your words. Pause and take additional breaths as needed.

Mouth stretch. Open and close your mouth five times, stretching your mouth as much as possible.

Wide smile. Smile five times, stretching your lips back as far as possible.

Nonsense syllables. Smile widely and say "ma, ma, me, me" and "ma, me, mi, mo."

Even syllables. Try saying "puh, puh, puh" ten times. Repeat each syllable evenly and slowly. Use a metronome if you have one. Pronounce the syllables quickly and evenly. Repeat the instructions above using "tah, tah, tah," then "kuh, kuh, kuh," and finally "puh, tuh, kuh," ten times each.

Tongue out. Stick your tongue out five times. Make it come straight out of your mouth.

Tongue push-ups. Stick out your tongue and push it against the back of a spoon. Repeat five times.

Tongue movement. Move your tongue from side to side and back and forth five times.

Kiss. Pucker your lips as if to kiss a child five times. (Then kiss your caregiver five times!)

Swallowing Problems

Swallowing difficulties, or *dysphagia,* may be more serious than speech problems. Dysphagia may cause life-threatening *aspiration,* the passage of food or drink into the airways. Swallowing seems like a simple enough task, but it's actually quite complicated, involving many nerves and muscles that act simultaneously. PD may affect regions of the brain that detect the presence of food in the mouth or throat, or it may affect the muscles involved in swallowing.

Some people with swallowing problems are unable to feel food or liquid going down the wrong way or getting stuck in the throat. Thus, liquid can enter the air pipe, which may in turn cause an infection, even pneumonia. Choking on food lodged in the airway can be fatal.

Poor nutrition can result from eating difficulties, as can avoidance of social situations.

Signs of Swallowing Problems

Some people with PD have swallowing difficulties and aren't even aware of it. If you or someone you love has PD, be on the lookout for the signs listed below and seek help quickly.

- Coughing or throat clearing during or after a meal
- Being awakened by coughing
- Experiencing changes in voice quality, especially making a wet or gurgling sound
- Requiring an exceptionally long time to eat a meal
- Having noticeable difficulty eating
- Experiencing weight loss or dehydration
- Requiring beverages to wash down foods

- Noticing that food or liquid gets stuck in the throat or goes down the wrong way
- Having a fever
- Showing signs of pneumonia

When you go in for diagnosis, a speech pathologist will evaluate your swallowing as you eat various foods and beverages. He or she may have you swallow barium and then do an X-ray study to see the muscles and other structures involved in swallowing. The pathologist will then develop an individualized program for you. Your program may include instructions to eat when you are in an "on" period, that is, when your medications are providing maximum benefit and it is easier to swallow.

Dealing with Vision Changes

It is not uncommon for people with PD to experience vision changes. Some say their vision is blurred. Others have problems focusing and reading. Still others report that their "eyes are bothering" them. Often people with PD visit their eye doctors seeking stronger glasses or contacts, only to be told their corrected vision is perfect.

Another common vision problem is dry eyes. This may be a side effect of some anti-Parkinson medications. More often, it is caused by disease-related infrequent blinking. Over-the-counter eye drops called "artificial tears" usually solve this problem.

Some people with PD complain of eye-muscle fatigue. Often the fatigue is worse on one side, causing double vision. Anticholinergics may aggravate these and other eye problems.

If you experience eye problems, talk with your doctor about a possible change needed in your medication.

Can you drive if you have PD? For many, driving represents freedom and independence. Losing that independence can lead to isolation and depression for those not ready to cope with this change in their lives.

Early in your disease when your symptoms are mild, you will likely still be able to drive. However, as symptoms progress, driving safely may no longer be possible because of muscle rigidity and impaired coordination. Your driving could endanger you, your passengers, and others on the road.

If you have questions about your ability to continue driving, talk with your doctor. Prepare for the time when you can no longer drive by familiarizing yourself with your area's public transportation, taxicabs, and vans for senior citizens and people with disabilities. And don't hesitate to call upon friends and family who have asked, "How can I help?"

For those whose disease is well controlled, driving may continue to be a pleasure. If you consider yourself still able to drive safely, follow these commonsense tips:

- Don't drive if you feel fatigued or unstable.

- Don't drive if you have consumed any alcohol. A small amount of alcohol may impair even healthy drivers. Drinking alcohol may also interfere with or dangerously interact with medications. Talk with your doctor about alcoholic beverages and your medications.

- Avoid driving after sunset. Even healthy adults have difficulty seeing well in the dark.

Dealing with Sexuality Issues

Sexual desire and sexual performance are highly individual. Later in life, some men and women have less sexual desire. For some older men, sexual dysfunction—especially difficulty achieving and maintaining an erection—is a problem. After menopause, some women experience a marked decrease in sexual desire. For most, PD comes later in life and coincides with a decline in sexual interest and activity.

Many men and women, however, remain sexually interested and active well into their later years. We are sexual beings. Sexual relationships fill basic biological needs. Moreover, a satisfying sexual relationship may fulfill our need for intimacy, closeness, touch, and pleasure. It may help us release tension and connect with another human being.

Little information is available about the impact of PD on sexuality. Research shows that PD affects the autonomic nervous system. As a result, the disease affects one's response to sexual stimulation. In addition, PD inhibits agility and the capacity to move freely—impairing your ability to express emotions, causing incontinence and bowel problems, and shrinking unused muscles. Many anti-Parkinson drugs decrease sexual desire and diminish sexual functioning. Less commonly, anti-Parkinson dopamine medications result in *hypersexuality*—mild to severe increases in sexual desire and interest accompanied by vivid dreams and sleep disturbances.

The changes that men experience in sexual function may be related as much to aging as they are to PD. The male sex hormone testosterone begins diminishing after age twenty-five. By age fifty, achieving an erection takes two to three times longer than at age thirty-five or forty. Often, a full erection cannot be achieved until just before climax. Not only does it take longer to get an erection, but the erection may disappear quickly after orgasm. As arteries narrow with aging, blood flow to the penis is decreased or blocked, making erection difficult or impossible.

In men with PD, changes in the autonomic nervous system may interfere with the brain's signal to the penis for erection. Drugs taken for PD or other health problems sometimes hamper erection. Bladder and bowel problems, especially incontinence, may also affect sexual function.

Erection difficulties and other sexual problems can have a huge impact on a man's self-concept. Culturally, sexual prowess is an indicator of manhood. The inability to achieve and maintain an erection and "perform" sexually can be the ultimate humiliation. For men with PD who have already been robbed of many traditional male roles, sexuality problems often erode self-esteem as well.

Most women with PD have undergone or are undergoing menopause. This major life change causes the clitoris to shrink, decreases normal lubrication in the vagina, and makes the vaginal walls thinner and less elastic, which can make intercourse painful or less satisfying. In addition, some women experience changes in sexual desire with menopause. Some have more desire, while others have less or almost none.

Fluctuations in the female hormones progesterone and estrogen may make some anti-Parkinson medications work less effectively or quit working altogether. For most women, the problems occur just before menses every month. Postmenopausal women, too, may experience hormone fluctuations that produce similar problems with anti-Parkinson medications.

Some women have difficulty experiencing orgasms. PD impedes autonomic nerve responses and muscle movement, both important in sexual response. Drugs for PD and other health problems sometimes make achieving orgasm problematic. As with men, bowel and bladder problems may also negatively affect sexual desire and functioning. On an emotional level, PD may attack a woman's belief in her femininity. As the disease progresses, a woman possibly sees herself as less attractive, less desirable, and less able to be a fulfilling sexual partner.

Suggestions for Being Sexual

There are many things you and your partner can do to improve your sex life.

Get your disease under control. A balanced drug regimen is the best treatment for PD symptoms that affect sexuality. In addition, it is important to employ all the self-help strategies you can to lessen the impact of your symptoms on your sexuality, including exercising regularly, getting enough rest, managing stress, and eating a well-balanced diet.

Try satin sheets. They make turning over in bed easier and can improve agility.

Plan sex for "on" times. Some people object to planning sexual activity, claiming it takes the spontaneity out of sex. However, spontaneity is not necessary for sexual satisfaction. Planning seduction—and timing it so that it coincides with times when your anti-Parkinson drugs are most effective—may actually increase anticipation and sexual pleasure.

Renew romance. Couples who have been together for a long time perhaps have lost the romance and passion of their early years. PD may complicate this further, especially as the disease progresses. For someone with PD, the symptoms and physical limitations often make it difficult to feel sexual. In the case of an exhausted caregiver, sexual activity is probably the last thing on his or her mind. Some lucky couples find that the challenges of PD bring them even closer together. Others are not so fortunate.

Make time for romance. A candlelight dinner, a single rose, sultry music, dancing in the moonlight—all can set the stage for renewed intimacy.

Talk about it. Honest communication is the key factor to a mutually satisfying relationship, regardless of age or physical condition. Ask for what you need sexually.

Get help. All of us carry some psychological issues concerning sex. Combine these with a chronic illness, and the result may prove disastrous. If your efforts to improve your communication and your sex life aren't enough, consider talking with a mental-health therapist. A skilled therapist can often help couples work through even the most difficult issues.

Incontinence and Constipation

Some Parkinson's patients experience bladder problems. As a disorder of the nervous system, PD may cause overactive bladder. This means you may feel an urgency to urinate more frequently. When this occurs during the night, it can disrupt sleep. Some patients report slowness in starting the flow of urine. If you have incontinence problems, here are several steps you can take.

- *Get evaluated by a urologist.* It's the only way to find out what is causing the problem.

- *Ask about changing medications.* Sometimes bowel and bladder problems are side effects of medications.

- *Practice Kegel exercises for women.* Ask your doctor about these exercises, which may improve muscle tone in the vagina, control the urinary outlet, and help prevent urine leakage. To do Kegel exercises, squeeze and release the muscles in the vaginal area as if to stop the flow of urine. You can practice Kegels throughout the day—while driving, sitting, or lying down.

- *Drink plenty of water.* Drink six to eight glasses of water or juice daily (throughout the day, not all at once) to improve overall health and regularity.

- *Limit beverages at night.*

- *Try grapefruit juice and coffee.* Both stimulate urination to help you empty your bladder.

- *Talk to your doctor about water pills.* Taking a diuretic medication in the morning may help prevent incontinence.

- *Don't wait until you feel the urge to urinate.* Women in particular have been taught to "hold it" rather than urinating when the urge strikes. Take every opportunity to empty your bladder.

- *Urinate before sexual activity.* It will help prevent urine spillage during climax.

- *Eat roughage.* If constipation is a problem, eat lots of fiber, such as found in fruits, vegetables, and bran.

- *Exercise regularly.* It helps relieve constipation and improves overall physical and mental health.

Dealing with Dizziness and Fainting

Some people with PD suffer from low blood pressure (*orthostatic hypotension*). If your blood pressure is extremely low, you may experience dizziness, fainting, fatigue, unsteadiness, or slowing of mental processes. It is often most noticeable when you rise from a sitting or lying position. The following tips may be helpful:

Do a medication check. Talk with your doctor about stopping any unnecessary medications. Low blood pressure can be a side effect of nearly all anti-Parkinson drugs. Also talk to your physician about medications that may help with low blood pressure.

Drink water. Drink at least six glasses a day to replenish body fluids.

Try wearing thigh-high elastic stockings. They can help prevent pooling of blood in the lower legs.

Take care when rising from a sitting or lying position. Take your time and get up slowly. Fatigue and sitting for long periods in a warm bath or another warm environment are definitely aggravating factors. Have someone at your side when you stand up. Sit or lie down immediately if you begin to feel the symptoms.

Calming Restless Legs

Restless leg syndrome (RLS) is a motor-movement disorder that creates uncomfortable sensations in the legs. Some people describe RLS as feeling like a pulling, tingling, or aching in the legs. Others describe a need to move their legs. The exact cause of the disorder is not known.

RLS comes on when one is inactive, with symptoms usually becoming worse during sleep. RLS episodes in one or both legs may disturb your sleep. Even when not fully awakened by the disorder, a person with RLS might get up in the morning feeling unrested.

Although rubbing or moving the legs immediately after experiencing the sensation occasionally relieves the discomfort, it usually returns within seconds. If you have RLS, ask your doctor if medication might help. Some people obtain relief from a combination of carbidopa and levodopa; others report good results with one of the dopamine agonists. Sometimes a hot, soothing bath helps.

Staying Safe and Comfortable at Home

More than 90 percent of people with PD live at home with loved ones. Home is where most of us feel comfortable and safe. Home can become a dangerous place, however, if necessary adaptations aren't made to accommodate the changes caused by PD. (See Resources for information about companies that offer adaptive aids.)

Preventing Falls

Falls are the most common cause of accidental injury in the home. Anyone who is ill, injured, frail, or elderly is especially at risk. Many older people with PD have lost calcium in their bones, making them even more vulnerable to serious injury from falling. A few simple changes around the house can help ensure safety.

Make walkways safe. Tack down or remove loose carpets and throw rugs. Remove raised doorsills. Move furniture out of walkways. Make sure all furniture with sharp edges or corners is removed. Install handrails adjacent to entryways and in hallways. Take breakable objects out of harm's way.

Make stairs safe. Stairways should have sturdy railings. Repair cracked steps, loose handrails, and other problem areas that may cause falls. Install colored strips of tape on steps to make their edges more visible.

Increase lighting. Install soft, nonglare 100-watt bulbs above staircases and 75-watt bulbs in hallways. Shade bulbs to prevent excess glare. Place night lights where appropriate. Install motion-activated lights that turn on when someone passes a sensor.

Make bathrooms safe. Install grab bars next to the toilet and in the shower and bathtub. Use nonskid rubber mats in the shower and bathtub. Make sure the toilet is the right height. Raised toilet seats, available at home-care supply stores, makes rising from the toilet easier and safer.

Making Meals Enjoyable

People with PD often eat slowly and have difficulty chewing and swallowing—all of which can make mealtimes frustrating. Lack of coordination often makes cooking meals difficult, even dangerous. A few adaptations will help you prepare and enjoy meals once again.

Take all the time you need. Accept the fact that it will take longer for you to cook and eat. Take your time. Chew your food thoroughly. If your food gets cold, use an electric warming tray. Others at your table can use the time to sit and enjoy one another's company.

Have someone cut your meat. Handling a knife may be a problem. Ask someone to cut your meat into bite-size pieces.

Choose utensils that work. Use a spoon instead of a fork if it makes eating less awkward for you. Home-health-aid stores offer special utensils with thicker handles that are easier to grasp than regular ones.

Drink through a straw. Tremors may make drinking difficult. A flexible straw should help.

Choose large-handled mugs, especially if grasping is difficult.

Alter the texture. Try preparing your food in a food processor or blender. Thick soups or stews are often easier to eat than other types of food.

Eat smaller meals more often. It is easier to digest smaller amounts of food. Smaller, more frequent meals will also help you maintain a constant supply of energy throughout the day. Try eating a light breakfast, a mid-morning snack, a light lunch, a midafternoon snack, a moderate dinner, and a light meal later in the evening (but at least an hour before bedtime).

Use helpful kitchen aids. Cooking may be easier if you use such kitchen aids as jar openers, cutting boards with suction cups and lips to keep food from slipping off, "reachers" to grasp items in cupboards or pick up dropped items, and pot stabilizers to keep pots and pans from sliding off the stove. Electric can openers are also convenient. Cooking in a microwave oven might be safer and more suitable than using a stove or a conventional oven.

Dressing/Grooming Made Easier

PD may impair the fine motor coordination and strength required for dressing and grooming. A few adaptations can help you maintain your independence in these very personal tasks.

Wear shoes with Velcro strips instead of laces. Or buy elastic shoelaces that are permanently tied and simply slip your shoes on and off.

Replace buttons with zippers or other fasteners that are easier to use. Large zipper pulls or rings make opening and closing garments easier. For blouse or shirt cuffs, sew on buttons with elastic thread that allows you to slip your hand through without unbuttoning.

Choose loose, stretchy clothing. It's easier to get on and off.

Enlarge armholes. If you have PD, coat sleeves may be too narrow to get your arm into easily. Have a tailor widen the armholes by two inches so that you may put on your coat without assistance.

Try a front-closing bra. They are usually easier to fasten than back-closing bras.

Use a long-handled shoehorn and a sock donner. They may prevent straining when you put on socks and shoes.

Turn up the heat. The fewer clothes the better for many people with PD. Turn the heat up a bit so that you don't have to wear layers of clothes.

Use an electric shaver to avoid cuts from razors. Holders for electric razors are also available, if needed.

Other Helpful Aids

Books on tape. They provide excellent entertainment, especially for someone with tired eyes.

Bed pulls. Bed pulls attached to the sides or the ends of your bed frame make it easier for you to turn over in bed and to get into or out of bed. You can buy them, or make your own by braiding three pieces of fabric together and attaching large wooden curtain rings on the ends as handles. They should be long enough so that you can reach them when you're lying down.

Trapeze. A triangular handle may be installed over the head of your bed to make it easier to change positions.

Urinals. Kept within easy reach, they can eliminate nighttime walks to the bathroom.

Wedge cushions. These may make sitting up in bed easier.

Bed rails. To help you turn over and get out of bed, bed rails may be installed on the wall near your bed or attached to your bed frame.

Make the bathroom more user-friendly. Try a suction nailbrush to make grooming easier. It may be secured to the tub. Use soap on a rope. This keeps soap conveniently within reach. Try a long-handled brush or sponge for bathing. Replace tub faucet handles. Single-arm control levers are easier to operate. A tub seat or shower chair will allow you to sit while bathing. A handheld shower hose can be detached from the shower head and you can use it sitting down, if you like. Usually these devices have different settings that regulate the water pressure and pattern.

Making Travel Easier

PD may make travel more difficult, but not impossible. If you love to travel, don't give it up. With a little help, travel can still be part of your life. You'll learn that by planning ahead, you can still travel and maintain optimal comfort.

- *Travel with a companion.* This will make your trip easier and, in many cases, more fun.

- *Ask for help.* Although it is important to be as independent as possible, it is equally important to ask for help when you need it and let people know exactly what assistance you require. Employees in the travel and hospitality industries are accustomed to providing help for their customers. You can arrange in advance to board a plane before the other passengers and to be assisted (with a wheelchair if necessary) if you have to change planes. Bellhops can handle your luggage. Waiters are happy to cut your meat in the kitchen.

- *Take extra medication.* Take copies of your prescriptions. Be sure to carry these on board rather than checking them with your baggage.

- *Wear a Medic-Alert bracelet.* It will give essential information to medical personnel in the event of an emergency.

9

Caring for Caregivers

When your partner, parent, or someone you love develops PD, he or she isn't the only one affected. Everyone in the family is impacted by the disease, especially caregivers.

Caregiving is difficult—emotionally, spiritually, and physically. Though caregiving is an expression of love, it is also frustrating, lonely, isolating, and at times overwhelming, even for the strongest and most dedicated people. This chapter is for caregivers, the foot soldiers in the fight against PD.

At its best, caregiving is a mutual relationship. True, one partner may give more than the other. A health crisis such as PD may actually strengthen the bonds and intimacy a couple shares. At its worst, caregiving may breed resentment and anger between caregiver and patient. Both may feel overwhelmed but reluctant to ask for outside help. As more demands are placed on the caregiver and the roles of each person change, the relationship may be strained to the breaking point.

Coping with Emotional Challenges

Learning that your partner or another loved one has PD means changing the lifestyle you have shared and embarking on a way of life you're not prepared for. It means a future that is uncertain in many respects and all too certain in others. Confusing and conflicting feelings are likely to come up—anger, sadness, hopelessness, resentment—and guilt for *having* those feelings.

Here are some examples of the feelings expressed by caregivers:

Anger. "Sometimes I feel trapped. I struggle with feelings of anger and guilt."

Sadness. "I've lost a healthy spouse to a chronic, disabling, incurable disease. We had so much to look forward to."

Loneliness. "Everybody wants to know how he's feeling. No one even asks about me."

Guilt. "I sometimes feel ashamed of my feelings."

Resentment. "I didn't ask for this burden. Why me?"

Hopelessness. "Everything changes, and you realize your lives will never be the same again."

Loss of intimacy. "We don't communicate well. We're less intimate. How do I explain that I'm scared and feel deprived?"

All too often, in caring for someone with PD, your needs and feelings take second place. There is much that you can do, however, to cope with the negative aspects of caregiving.

Give yourself permission to feel your feelings. Feelings are neither good nor bad. They're just feelings. Accept that many so-called negative feelings such as sadness, anger, frustration, guilt, and resentment are all part of caregiving. Allow yourself to recognize all your feelings and let go of your guilt.

Learn effective ways to release difficult emotions. Exercising, talking with supportive friends and family members, meditating, writing in your journal, and utilizing stress-reduction techniques are all good ways to let go of negative feelings. *Channel your feelings into constructive behavior.* You're feeling angry and frustrated. You call the doctor, yell, and hang up. Or you scream at your children, kick the dog, or smash an antique vase. None of these is an effective coping strategy. Your feelings aren't the problem. It's how you act on those feelings that counts. Try rechanneling your anger and frustration into forming a support group for caregivers, finding the community services you need, or raising money for PD research.

Recognize and get help for depression. The losses associated with PD and the demands placed on you may cause you to sink into depression. Seek professional help.

Talk about your feelings. Talk with your doctor, your loved one, your friends, your family, members of your PD support group—anyone who will care and understand—about your feelings.

Put your anger where it belongs. Anger, resentment, and blaming can spill over onto your partner and to other friends and family members. Instead, get angry with the disease. Give yourself permission to blame the illness for your troubles. It frees you from blaming yourself or your partner for circumstances that are beyond your control.

Accept that to give is also to receive. There are many gifts you get back as a caregiver, including feelings of accomplishment, pride, joy, relief, love, and commitment.

Find something to do while you allow your partner the time to accomplish those things he or she can still do. Listen to music, read, knit, or answer mail so you don't feel as though you are wasting time.

Learn relaxation techniques. Meditation, progressive relaxation, visualization, and biofeedback may help.

Practice positive self-talk. Instead of telling yourself how bad things are, tell yourself that you can do this, that you have successfully faced many challenges before. Know that others are worse off than you and that you have much to be grateful for.

Become involved in a support group. If your community doesn't have a caregiver support group, start one. Get help from your doctor, a hospital social worker, or a mental-health agency. Look for a caregiver community online.

Don't be afraid to laugh. Every difficult situation has its humor. Taking a lighter approach may reduce stress and help you face difficult times.

Take time for yourself. You deserve to have pleasure and joy in your life. You must nourish yourself, take time for yourself, and care for yourself. If you want to be there for your loved one, you must give yourself time-outs to pursue other interests and enjoy other relationships. Ask family and friends if they can take over caregiving duties occasionally so that you may have a break. See a movie, visit a friend, or take up a hobby.

Mobilize friends and family to help. Often we think we should do everything ourselves. However, caring for someone with a chronic illness is oftentimes overwhelming. Let others know how they can help and gratefully accept their assistance.

Bring in some paid help. If you don't have family support, consider hiring an in-home caregiver or taking your loved one to a daytime care program.

Adjust your expectations. Life won't be "normal" no matter how much you want it to be. Don't insist on normalcy. Some chores such as dusting, vacuuming, cleaning, and yard work may have to be cut back, eliminated, or delegated to someone else. Life doesn't have to be perfect.

Handling a Spiritual Crisis

For many caregivers, spirituality provides the strength needed to face the challenges of PD. But the rigors of caregiving may bring on a spiritual crisis for both the caregiver and the person with PD.

Instead of the joys of leisure and retirement, you both now face the uncertainty of a chronic disease. You may ask, "Why me?" You sometimes think your Higher Power has let you down. Or perhaps you feel guilty because you think it is a sin to be angry with God. You may even begin to lose your faith.

"Why do bad things happen to good people?" you may ask. Few explanations can make sense of such things. Perhaps it makes more sense to ask, "How will I respond?" and "What will I do now?"

If you find your spirituality is waning, find someone to help. Your pastor, rabbi, counselor, or another trusted person can help you gain new perspectives on your situation.

Here are some suggestions for facing your spiritual challenges:

Accept that you are not in control. It is difficult for most of us to acknowledge that we have little control over many aspects of our lives. Once you accept that fact, you can surrender what you can't control and tackle the challenges where you can make a difference.

Find pleasure in small wonders. Take time to appreciate a beautiful sunset, a blooming flower, the changing seasons, the laughter of a child.

Keep a grateful journal. Take time each day to write down five things for which you are grateful. They can be as small as the taste of a cup of coffee or as grand as your gratitude for freedom. Record all your grateful observations in your journal.

Reconnect with your spiritual self. Take time each day to meditate, pray, or otherwise connect with that quiet place inside and your higher spiritual power.

Spend time in nature. For many people, walking in the woods is more spiritual than spending time in a place of worship. Connecting with nature can awaken you to the miracle that is life.

Change your perspective on caregiving. Instead of seeing caregiving as a burden you must bear, look at it as an opportunity to grow and learn.

See yourself as strong and capable. Take time each day to visualize yourself competently handling all the challenges you face. Try using affirmations such as "I capably handle all the challenges I am presented with" or "I have all the resources I need to handle any situation."

Facing the Physical Challenges

PD challenges a caregiver physically. Suddenly, you are faced not only with caring for your ill partner but also with assuming many of his or her customary tasks. A husband, for instance, who chopped wood and took care of the yard work before becoming ill may now not be able to do that work. A wife who previously did the cooking, shopping, and housecleaning may have to turn over those tasks to her husband.

Often, caregiving means being pushed physically beyond your endurance. For example, you hurriedly grab a bite to eat in the kitchen. You are worn out from being awakened at night by a partner who is restless from PD symptoms or medications. Your back aches from lifting and moving your partner.

It is not uncommon for caregivers to become ill themselves. Research has demonstrated that stress contributes to a host of ailments, including high blood pressure, ulcers, depression and anxiety, and heart disease. To cope with the physical, mental, and emotional challenges of caregiving, you must take care of yourself physically. Here are some tips.

Manage stress. Try humor, exercise, and relaxation techniques to manage the stress in your life.

Exercise regularly. Research shows that keeping physically fit helps reduce the emotional and physical strain. It may also make you stronger and better able to meet the physical demands of caregiving, such as helping a person move from a bed to a wheelchair.

Avoid excessive alcohol. Because it is a depressant, alcohol won't help you cope with your situation. If you find yourself turning to alcohol or other drugs to cope, get help fast.

Eat a well-balanced diet. A good diet is important for you, too. Eat plenty of whole grains, fruits, and vegetables. Drink six to eight glasses of water per day. Reduce fat, caffeine, alcohol, refined sugar, and salt.

Get plenty of rest. Lack of rest is a major contributor to depression and exhaustion. People with PD are often erratic sleepers. They may thrash about with vivid dreams, wake frequently, or talk in their sleep, leaving you sleepless and exhausted. As difficult as it may be to accept, perhaps it is time to consider sleeping in separate bedrooms or at least in separate beds.

Learn proper moving, lifting, and transferring techniques. Your loved one may feel humiliated and embarrassed to need assistance moving. However, as the disease progresses, it often becomes necessary for the caregiver to help the person with PD get into or out of chairs or bed. Using proper body mechanics and the right techniques and equipment may help maintain the ill person's dignity and prevent injuries. Talk with your loved one's doctor or physical therapist about the best lifting and moving techniques.

- Encourage your loved one to move as independently as possible.
- Allow plenty of time for moving.
- Move the person from his or her strongest side.
- Think safety to avoid falls. Check personal equipment such as wheelchairs and walkers before using. Lock side rails on beds. Use brakes on wheels of beds, shower chairs, wheelchairs, and commodes.
- Use the right equipment. Safety belts, lifts, and other aids can make lifting easier for you and the person you're moving.
- Use good body mechanics when assisting someone:
  - Use your legs rather than your back.
  - Spread your legs to give yourself a wide base of support.
  - Move your whole body rather than just bending or twisting.
  - Keep the person close to you.
  - Avoid jerky movements and lifting whenever possible. Instead, use rolling, pivoting, or sliding to move the person.
  - Get help when you need it.

Getting Help

As PD progresses, so do the demands placed on a caregiver. Many try to shoulder all the emotional and physical burdens alone. Even the best caregiver, for a variety of reasons, may no longer be able to continue caring for his or her loved one alone. Where can you find help?

Friends and family. Let others know exactly what kind of help you need. Perhaps you can work out a schedule so that a relative or friend can stay with your loved one or take him or her for an outing to give you a break.

Your place of worship. Religious communities can be invaluable sources of support. Depending on the size and the level of organization, religious communities offer everything from prayer support and home-cooked meals to full-fledged senior programs and adult day care.

Meals on Wheels. If cooking meals becomes difficult on top of all your other responsibilities, social-service programs such as Meals on Wheels will deliver hot meals to your home at little or no expense to you.

Community services. Check your state's Area Office on Aging for a list of the services offered in your community. Also, look in your local phone book under "community services" and "senior services."

Home-care services. These provide either skilled nursing care prescribed by a physician or respite/support services for personal care and household chores. Be sure to shop around and investigate credentials before selecting a home-care agency or an individual to provide these services. You'll want to know

- about their experience working with people with PD.

- whether they are licensed and bonded.

- what references they can offer (be sure to check them).

- the fees charged. (Check with your insurance plan to see if any of the services is covered.)

Financial Help

PD can take a high financial toll. As soon as your loved one receives a diagnosis of PD, it is important to begin planning. Since each family's financial situation is different, no single formula works for everyone. The key is to plan as far ahead as possible to avoid having to react in a crisis and make poor decisions.

Take a realistic look at your financial situation. Cut down on unnecessary expenditures. If needed, hire a financial consultant, an accountant, or a lawyer to help. Legal Aid or Consumer Credit Counseling provides help at no cost if you meet income-eligibility requirements.

Thoroughly review your health insurance. What is covered? What is not covered? What is the maximum lifetime benefit? Does the policy cover long-term care? (Note: Medicare does not cover long-term nursing costs.) Will it cover in-home health services? If you don't have health insurance, many states now have insurance pools for those who meet income requirements.

Set up a budget. Be sure to include estimates for medications, doctor visits, and hospitalization not covered by your insurance.

Explore ways to maintain your family's income and still function as caregiver. Can you work out of your home, for example, or practice your profession as an independent contractor instead of an employee?

Contact Social Security. The staff will tell you about your benefits and eligibility requirements. Phone numbers are listed in the government section of your phone book, or look online at www.ssa.gov.

Contact Medicare. The specialists at Medicare can help you understand what Medicare does and does not cover. Check online at www.medicare.gov or look in the government section of your phone book. Also, under "disability services" in the phone book, look for Centers for Independent Living, or check online at www.ilru.org. These centers provide assistance for seniors and people who are disabled, including job counseling and housing assistance.

Get tax help. Provisions in the IRS tax code allow you to deduct medical expenses, including durable medical equipment and modifications to your home or automobile. At present, you may deduct costs for doctors, drugs, equipment, and treatment or therapies that exceed 7.5 percent of your adjusted gross income. Eligible home modifications include ramps, guardrails, and widened doorways. Talk with your accountant or tax adviser about how to make the most of these tax deductions.

Living Will and Durable Power of Attorney

Planned instructions—advance directives—give your loved one the power to govern medical, financial, and other decisions in the event you become incapable of making them. Advance directives, which relieve the caregiver and other family members of having to make potentially agonizing decisions, need not cost any money to prepare.

Living Will

A living will is an advance directive on treatment to be given if and when a patient is no longer mentally or physically capable of making such decisions. In effect, a living will is a statement of a person's desire to die with dignity. It usually expresses the individual's wish that no extraordinary life-sustaining measures be taken. An attorney may draw up a living will. You might be able to use standard forms or make your own, but first check your state laws.

Durable Power of Attorney

This document identifies a person (often a partner-caregiver) to act as the patient's agent if he or she becomes incapacitated. Be sure to investigate your state's laws regarding durable power of attorney. Some states require special witnesses or restrict who can be appointed agent.

Long-Term Care: Making Difficult Decisions

As mentioned, most people with PD live at home. For some, complications from the disease or other health problems eventually make this impossible. Deciding to place a loved one in a care home or nursing home can be extremely difficult for caregivers and their families. You may be torn by your loved one's resistance to leaving home and your need for help.

Let's face it, there's no place like home. In the best of all worlds, all of us would end our days in our homes surrounded by loved ones and caregivers with inexhaustible reserves of energy, patience, and time. This isn't always possible, however. As a caregiver, perhaps you are facing health problems of your own. Other family members may have more energy for caregiving but much less time.

Moreover, it may not be financially feasible to continue caregiving at home, even though it is less expensive than a care facility. Financial resources to hire the extra help that would make home care possible are hard to find. Medicaid, for instance, which is available to low-income families, pays few home-care costs but covers full-time nursing-home costs.

Even when you can afford at-home care or day care, PD patients with mental alterations often feel threatened by any change. They may resist new caregivers, refuse to attend day-care programs, or lash out at their partner-caregivers. Over time, disease progression and mobility impairment can make at-home care impossible and even dangerous.

Here are some suggestions for helping with the transition from at-home care to full-time placement:

Plan ahead. Talk with your loved one honestly about the need for care facilities in the future. If possible, visit facilities and make choices before such care is necessary. For some people, it is impossible to face the impending loss of their independence and take these steps. This leaves the caregiver to make these decisions, often alone, and sometimes with criticism from other family members.

Work with your primary-care doctor. Your doctor will determine what level of care is needed for your loved one. It is also likely that your doctor has established relationships with one or more care facilities in your area. Ask him or her for recommendations.

Check with your Area Office on Aging. This agency publishes a guide to nursing homes that contains basic information you will need to make an informed choice.

Ask for a Medicare assessment. Call your local Medicare office and ask for a nursing-home admission review. Medicare personnel will determine whether your loved one qualifies for coverage in a skilled-care facility. If you are under your state's insurance plan, staff members for that program can determine eligibility.

Treat the facility as your loved one's home. Once your loved one has been moved to a care facility, make it feel homey. Bring personal items to make the room feel familiar. A photograph of your partner at a young age will help caregivers at the facility remember that your loved one was once youthful and independent.

Give it time. Adjustment to a new place is always challenging. If your loved one has memory problems, avoid taking him or her for drives or visits home for at least six weeks or until he or she has accepted the facility as a new home. It may be heart-wrenching to persuade a confused loved one to go back to the care facility after a visit home.

Develop good relationships. Remember that you and your family should strive for a cordial relationship with the care-facility personnel. Avoid being hypercritical. No matter how good the care facility, it is not home. Don't misplace your guilt by becoming angry with the facility.

Get a feel for the place. Make a habit of visiting the facility at different times of the day. Attend an activity. Eat a meal there. Try not to make snap decisions about the facility, especially during the first few weeks of adjustment.

To determine whether your loved one is receiving good care, ask yourself the following questions:

- How is your loved one doing compared with functioning at home?
- Is your loved one clean and dry?
- Is he or she encouraged to be as active as possible?
- Is he or she receiving the individualized care needed to support mobility, functioning, and personal dignity?
- Is your loved one receiving medications on time and in the correct dose?

If you have concerns, talk with the nurse in charge or the facility's administrator.

Make sure the staff understands the challenges of PD. Some staff may not have much experience caring for people with PD. Make sure, for instance, that they understand how important it is to administer medications exactly on time and to provide opportunities for exercise. If you need help educating the facility staff, talk with your doctor.

In Conclusion

Many scientific accomplishments have resulted in better treatments today for Parkinson's disease, and scientists are at work with new research. Some of this research focuses not only on better PD treatment but also on preventing and curing the disease. Because any potential new treatment must undergo painstaking scrutiny to determine potential harm as well as benefit, it is impossible to say how soon new treatments might be available. But efforts are under way.

We have much to be optimistic about—scientists are working diligently to unlock the secrets of Parkinson's disease. But, until researchers discover a more effective treatment or even a cure for PD, we must never give up hope. We must strive to stay independent and enjoy each day. The joy in life comes from inside each of us, and we must remain upbeat and hopeful, enjoying each day to the fullest.

Resources

American Parkinson Disease Association
135 Parkinson Avenue
Staten Island, NY 10305
Phone: 718-981-8001 / 800-223-2732
www.apdaparkinson.org

American Speech-Language-Hearing Association
2200 Research Boulevard
Rockville, MD 20850-3289
Phone: 301-296-5700
Members: 800-498-2071
Non-Member: 800-638-8255
TTY: 301-296-5650
www.asha.org

Bachmann-Strauss Dystonia & Parkinson Foundation
Mt. Sinai Medical Center
One Gustave L. Lev Place
P.O. Box 1490
Phone: 212-682-9900
www.dystonia-parkinsons.org

California Advocates for Nursing Home Reform
650 Harrison Street, 2nd Floor
San Francisco, CA 94107

Phone: 415-974-5171 / 800-474-1116
www.canhr.org

Family Caregiver Alliance
180 Montgomery Street, Suite 1100
San Francisco, CA 94104
Phone: 415-434-3388 / 800-445-8106
www.caregiver.org

Med Help International Parkinson's Disease Community
www.medhelp.org/forums/show/201

MedicAlert Foundation International
2323 Colorado Avenue
Turlock, CA 95382
Phone: 888-633-4298 / 209-668-3333 from outside the U.S.
www.medicalert.org

Michael J. Fox Foundation for Parkinson's Research
Church Street Station / P.O. Box 780
New York, NY 10008
Phone: 212-509-0995
www.michaeljfox.org

Movement Disorder Society
555 East Wells Street, Suite 1100
Milwaukee, WI 53202-3823
Phone: 414-276-2145
www.movementdisorders.org

National Institute of Neurological Disorders and Stroke
National Institutes of Health
NIH Neurological Institute
P.O. Box 5801
Bethesda, MD 20824
Phone: 301-496-5751 / 800-352-9424

TTY: 301-468-5981
www.ninds.nih.gov

National Parkinson Foundation
1501 N.W. 9th Avenue / Bob Hope Road
Miami, FL 33136-1494
Phone: 305-243-6666 / 800-327-4545
www.Parkinson.org

National Rehabilitation Information Center (NARIC)
8201 Corporate Drive, Suite 600
Landover, MD 20785
Phone: 301-459-5900 / 800-346-2742
TTY: 301-459-5984
www.naric.com

Parkinson's Action Network
1025 Vermont Avenue, NW, Suite 1120
Washington, DC 20005
Phone: 202-638-4101 / 800-850-4726
Fax: 202-638-7257
www.parkinsonsaction.org

Parkinson Alliance
P.O. Box 308
Kingston, NJ 08528
Phone: 609-688-0870 / 800-579-8440
www.parkinsonalliance.org

Parkinson's Disease Foundation
1359 Broadway, Suite 1509
New York, NY 10018
Phone: 212-923-4700 / 800-457-6676
www.pdf.org

PD Index—Directory of PD Information on the Internet
www.pdindex.org

Parkinson's Institute
1170 Morse Avenue
Sunnyvale, CA 94089
Phone: 408-734-2800 / 800-786-2958
www.thepi.org

Parkinson's Resource Organization
74-090 El Paseo Drive – Suite 102
Palm Desert, CA 92260
Phone: 760-773-5628
www.parkinsonsresource.org

Patterson Medical/Sammons Preston
1000 Remington Blvd., Suite 210
Bolingbrook, IL 60440
Phone: 800-323-5547
www.sammonspreston.com

Offers a selection of home health aids like special shower chairs, handgrips, grab bars, reacher sticks, sock and stocking aids, button-up and zipper pulls.

Wardrobe Wagon Special-Needs Clothing Store
555 Valley Road
West Orange, NJ 07052
Phone: 800-992-2737
www.wardrobewagon.com

WE MOVE (Worldwide Education & Awareness for Movement Disorders)
204 West 84th Street
New York, NY 10024
Phone: 212-875-8312
www.wemove.org

Glossary

A

Acetylcholine: A chemical that in the brain can act as a neurotransmitter. In Parkinson's disease, an imbalance can occur between dopamine and acetylcholine, causing some of the symptoms.

Agonist: A chemical substance or drug capable of activating a receptor site to induce a full or partial pharmacological response.

Aerobic Exercise: Various sustained exercises designed to stimulate and strengthen the body and the heart.

Amantadine (Symmetrel): An antiviral drug that can provide benefit for some features of Parkinson's disease in some people.

Anticholinergic: A drug that blocks the action of acetylcholine, useful mostly for tremor in PD patients.

Antioxidant: An agent that prevents the loss of oxygen in chemical reactions.

Anti-Parkinson Drugs: Drugs used to treat symptoms of Parkinson's disease.

Apoptosis: A death of cells by shrinking and disappearing, thought to be the way neurons are lost in the brain.

Aspiration: The act of inhaling fluid or a foreign body into the bronchial tubes and the lungs.

Autonomic Nervous System: The system of nerves that involuntarily control the functions of blood vessels, the heart, the bowel, and glands.

B

Basal Ganglia: Large clusters of nerve cells deep in the brain that coordinate motor commands.

Biofeedback: A relaxation technique in which people are taught to control some unconscious body functions such as blood pressure and heart rate.

Blood Brain Barrier: Thickly packed cells in brain blood vessels that prevent many substances from entering the brain.

Bradykinesia: A gradual loss of spontaneous movement.

Bromocriptine (Parlodel): A dopamine agonist used to treat symptoms of Parkinson's disease.

C

Carbidopa: A drug used with levodopa to block the breakdown of levodopa to dopamine so that sufficient amounts reach the brain.

Carbon Monoxide: A colorless, odorless, poisonous gas produced when carbon burns with insufficient air. Exposure considered a possible contributor to PD.

Caregiver: Someone who provides care for others who are unable to care for themselves.

CAT Scan: A computerized X-ray machine helpful in performing surgical procedures of the brain.

Clinical Psychologist: A specialist (usually not a medical doctor) who deals with the diagnosis and treatment of behavioral and personality disorders.

Combined Drug Therapy: Treating a disease by combining certain drugs in an attempt to improve the patient's condition.

COMT: An abbreviation for catechol-O-methyltransferase, one of the main enzymes responsible for the metabolism of levodopa into dopamine.

Corpus Striatum: A mass of gray matter deep in the brain thought to help regulate motor and sensory functions.

D

Debilitate: To weaken.

Dementia: A loss of intellectual abilities.

Demerol (Meperidine): A narcotic painkiller, which should be used with caution in people taking selegiline (Eldepryl).

Deprenyl (Eldepryl, Selegiline, Jumex): A monoamine-oxidase inhibitor used to treat Parkinson's disease. It blocks the enzyme monoamine oxidase B, which normally breaks down dopamine.

Depression: Feelings of helplessness, hopelessness, and despair, and possible thoughts of suicide.

Dietitian: A licensed person who is an expert in nutrition.

Disability: How an impairment affects ability to perform certain everyday functions.

Dopamine: A chemical messenger in the brain that transmits impulses from one nerve cell to another, and is deficient in brains of Parkinson's patients.

Dopamine Agonists: Anti-Parkinson drugs that stimulate receptors in the brain and mimic the effects of dopamine.

Dopamine Receptors: Sites on the brain neurons that are activated by dopamine and some of which are activated by dopamine agonist drugs.

Dopa Decarboxylase: The enzyme that can destroy levodopa.

Double Vision (Diplopia): A condition of vision in which a single object appears double.

Drug Holiday: A brief (3- to 14-day) withdrawal from carbidopa/levodopa therapy when the side effects outweigh the benefits.

Dyskinesia: Abnormal involuntary movements that can result from long-term use of levodopa.

Dysphagia: Difficulty swallowing.

Dystonia: Slow twisting involuntary movement, associated with forceful muscle contractions or spasms.

E

Endogenous Depression: Depression that is secondary to a biochemical imbalance in the brain.

Electrothermal: The method of heat used in a pallidotomy.

Endorphins: A group of natural substances in the brain that are released in response to stress or exercise and react with the brain's pain receptors to reduce the sensation of pain.

Environmental Toxins: Harmful substances in the environment that may prove to be a potential cause of PD.

Enzyme: A substance that stimulates or speeds up a specific chemical reaction.

Enzyme Inhibitors: Drugs that block the enzymes that destroy levodopa and dopamine.

Experimental: Not yet proven or available for general use.

F

Fetal Tissue Neurons: Neurons of human fetal origin that when carefully placed in the brain of PD patients could replace lost neurons.

Fibrosis: The formation of scar-like tissue.

Free Radicals: Toxic substances produced by all cells but which can cause irreversible loss of neurons in the brain.

Freezing: A temporary, involuntary inability to move.

G

Gait: Walking or ambulation.

Gene Therapy: A method using genes (sequences of DNA) to treat disease.

Generic Drugs: Nonproprietary drugs that can be sold without a brand name.

Glaucoma: Disorder of the eye characterized by increase of pressure within the eyeball.

Globus Pallidus: A part of the brain important to motor function, which is selectively destroyed in pallidotomy.

Guided Imagery: A method of stress reduction utilizing music or other relaxing sounds, allowing you to take a "mental vacation."

H

Half-Life: The time necessary for a drug taken into the body to lose one-half of its effectiveness.

Hallucination: Perception of objects with no reality, usually arising from a disorder of the nervous system.

Heroin: A morphine derivative that is a narcotic and addictive.

High Frequency Electrical Stimulation: A reversible procedure in which a particular part of the brain is temporarily stimulated by an electrical charge to reduce symptoms on the opposite side of the body.

Hydrotherapy: The use of water in the treatment of disease or injury such as soothing baths and whirlpools.

Hypokinetic Dysarthria: Slow, difficult, poorly articulated speech.

I

Idiopathic: A disease of unknown origin or without apparent cause.

Impotence: Inability of a man to produce an erection.

Incontinence: Inability to control bowel or bladder function, resulting in spilling of fecal matter or urine.

K

Kegel Exercises: A method of muscle strengthening for women to help reduce urinary incontinence.

L

Laboratory Grown Cell: Cells grown in a laboratory or test tube.

Levodopa (L-dopa): The generic name for Sinemet and Sinemet CR, the drug of choice for the treatment of Parkinson's disease.

Liver Failure: When the liver is no longer able to work and is destroyed by a drug or a medical condition.

Livido Reticularis: A red to purplish mottling of the skin often on the lower extremities, which is a rare side effect of amantadine.

M

Masklike Facies: A loss of facial expression as seen in some people with PD.

Meditation: To engage in extended thought or contemplation as a method of reducing stress.

Mesentary: A membrane that enfolds the bowel and attaches it to the gut wall.

Messenger: A cell or substance that transfers information about the brain.

Metabolism: The assimilation and processing of substances in the body such as food into energy, or the physical and chemical processes in an organism by which its substance is produced, maintained, and destroyed, making energy available.

Mirapex (Pramipexole): A dopamine agonist for treating symptoms of Parkinson's disease.

Mitochondria: Structures in cells that provide the energy for cellular activity.

Monoamine Oxidase Inhibitors: A general term for a group of drugs that inhibit the enzyme that oxidizes or breaks down dopamine.

Motor Fluctuations: The complications of the treatment of PD affecting the ability to move. Examples are wearing-off of dose, on-off phenomena, and dyskinesia.

Motor Performance: The ability and capacity to move about and to maneuver the body.

Motor System Disorder: A disorder that affects muscle or body movement.

MRI: Magnetic resonance imaging—new imaging radiological techniques important for surgical procedures on the brain.

MPTP: The abbreviation for 1-methyl-4-phenyl-1,2,3,6-tetra-hydropyridine, a heroin derivative that may produce a Parkinson's-like disease in humans and animals.

N

Neuroimmunophilin: A substance that stimulates the growth of damaged brain cells and nerves and appears to cause growth of damaged neurons.

Neuron: A cell that is specialized to generate and/or conduct impulses and to carry information from one part of the brain to another.

Neuroprotective Therapy: Drug therapy that may protect brain neurons from damage or reduce the rate of destruction.

Neurotransmitter: Any of several chemical substances that transmit nerve impulses in the brain.

O

Occupational Therapist: A specialist who provides therapy utilizing useful and creative activities to facilitate psychological or physical rehabilitation.

On-Off Attacks: A change in the patient's condition, with sometimes-rapid fluctuations between uncontrolled movements and normal movement. Probably caused by changes in the ability to respond to levodopa. ON—improvement in Parkinson signs and symptoms. OFF—the state of re-emergence of Parkinson signs and symptoms when the medication's effect has waned.

Orthostatic Hypotension: A decrease in blood pressure that, upon standing, can result in dizziness and fainting. May be a symptom of Parkinson's disease or a side effect of anti-Parkinson medications.

Oxidation: Free radicals react with nearby molecules in a process called oxidation. Oxidation is thought to cause damage to tissues, including neurons.

P

Pallidotomy: A surgical procedure in which a part of the brain called the globus pallidus is partly destroyed in order to improve symptoms of tremor, rigidity, and bradykinesia.

Parkinsonism: A term referring to a group of conditions that are characterized by four typical symptoms: rigidity, tremor, postural instability, and bradykinesia.

Patient Advocate: A spouse, partner, friend, or caregiver who understands your condition and can act on your behalf in decision making and making sure you are getting the best possible care.

Pergolide (Permax): A dopamine agonist for the treatment of Parkinson's disease symptoms.

Physical Therapy: Specialty designed to help regain strength, coordination, balance, walking, and endurance.

Pill Rolling: A characteristic type of tremor involving the thumb and forefinger in people with PD.

Postural Hypotension: A sudden drop in blood pressure when arising from a lying or seated position.

Postural Instability: Impaired balance and coordination, often causing patients to lean forward or backward and to fall easily.

Pramipexole (Mirapex): A dopamine agonist used in the treatment of PD symptoms.

R

Range of Motion (ROM): The extent a joint will move from full extension to full flexion.

Receptors: Sites in the brain that allow the attachment of certain drugs, making them active and able to produce the desired results.

Resting Tremor: Tremor of the limbs or body while the body is at rest.

Restless Legs: An uncomfortable feeling in the legs, worse at night; sensation of tingling or pulling of leg muscles.

Retroperitoneum: The deepest area in the gut containing the ureters.

Rigidity: A symptom of the disease in which muscles feel stiff and display resistance to movement even when another person tries to move the affected part of the body such as an arm.

Ropinirole (Requip): A dopamine agonist used in the treatment of PD symptoms.

S

Seborrhea: A skin eruption usually of the scalp or mid-face that is red and flaky and common in PD.

Seizure: Contortion of the body and involuntary muscle contractions caused by spontaneous discharges from the brain.

Selegiline (Eldepryl Deprenyl): An enzyme inhibitor used in treating Parkinson's disease.

Serotonin: An amine that occurs in nervous tissue and blood vessels and functions as a neurotransmitter.

Sinemet: A combination of carbidopa/levodopa prescribed to treat symptoms of Parkinson's disease.

Social Worker: A specialist who helps improve social conditions in the community for people in need of assistance and advice.

Speech Therapist: A specialist who helps restore language and who helps with cognitive and swallowing problems.

SSRIs: Selective serotonin re-uptake inhibitors such as Prozac. Some doctors advise caution using these drugs in patients on Deprenyl (selegeline) as rare interactions may occur.

Starter Therapy: Using a drug alone to begin treatment.

Stem Cells: A type of cell grown in the test tube that can generate other human cells. A development that will accelerate efforts to grow human tissue for transplantation.

Stereotactic Surgery: Surgical technique for operating deep in the brain using a stereotactic frame on the head, which along with advanced radiological procedures allows the transfer of a probe deep into the brain through a tiny hole in the skull.

Stressor: A stimulus causing stress.

Stroke: An abnormal neurological condition in which blood flow to part of the brain is interrupted, causing nerve damage.

Substantia Nigra: A movement control center in the brain where loss of dopamine-producing nerve cells triggers the symptoms of Parkinson's disease. Substantia nigra means "black substance," so-called because the cells in this area of the brain are dark.

Support Group: A group of people who meet regularly to support or sustain each other by discussing problems affecting them in common.

T

Thalamotomy: Surgical destruction of a group of cells in the thalamus to abolish tremor on the side of the body opposite the surgery.

Thalamus: A part of the brain that receives information from the basal ganglia (an interconnected cluster of cells that coordinate normal movement, made up in part by the substantia nigra, corpus striatum, and globus pallidum).

Tolcapone (Tasmar): One of the new enzyme inhibitors for the treatment of PD.

Tranquilizers: Various drugs that have a mildly sedative, calming, or muscle-relaxing effect.

Tremor: Rhythmic shaking, usually of the hand, but also of the leg, tongue, or jaw. Occurs at rest when caused by PD.

V

Voice Inflection: A change of pitch or tone of the voice.

Y

Yoga Exercises: A type of stretching exercises that can improve muscle flexibility and range of motion.

Young-Onset PD: People who develop idiopathic PD under forty years of age, well before the typical onset after age fifty. The progression of their disease is usually much slower.

Index

A

abdominal tenderness, 59
abnormal dreams, 53
accelerated aging, 14
acetylcholine (ACh), 54, 60
active exercises, 80
aerobic exercise, 71, 73
agitation, 53, 55, 59
akinesia, 64
Akineton, 54
alcohol use, 89
Alzheimer's disease and
    Parkinson's disease, 60
amantadine, 55
    side effects, 55
American Academy of
    Neurology (ANA), 57
American
    Speech-Language-Hearin
    g Association, 92
amino acid, 50, 57
amyotrophic lateral
    sclerosis, 13
anti-Parkinson's drugs, 16
anticholinergics, 53–55
    side effects, 54, 55
antidepressant drugs, 7, 50,
    57
antinausea drugs, 50

antioxidants, 14
antipsychotic (neuroleptic)
    drugs, 15, 50
antiviral medication, 55
anxiety, 55
Apokyn injection, 52
apomorphine, 52, 53
Artane, 54
arteriosclerosis, 15
attitude, 2
Azilect, 56, 57

B

balance impairment, 5, 67
battery pack, 66
behavioral changes, 53
benztropine mesylate, 54
biofeedback, 28
biperden, 54
blood-brain barrier, 48
blood pressure drugs, 50
blood sugar test distortion,
    52
blurred vision, 52, 54, 55
bradykinesia, 5, 48, 64
brain cells, 4
brain chemical, 54, 60
bromocriptine, 52
burning pain, 51

C

caffeine reduction, 27, 89
carbidopa, 48
care for caregivers, 109–122
causes of Parkinson's
    disease, 13–15
chest pain, 59
chewing problems, 8
chills, 59
cholinesterase inhibitor, 60
choosing the right doctor,
    40, 41
clinical psychologist, 39
Cogentin, 54
compulsive behaviors, 53
computed tomography (CT)
    scan, 16, 64, 67
COMT inhibitors, catechol-
    O-methyltransferase
    (COMT) inhibitors, 56–60
    side effects, 59, 60
Comtan, 49, 58
confusion, 54, 57, 59
constipation, 8, 55, 60, 101,
    102
coordination issues, 5
coping emotionally, 16–36
corrective exercises, 76
counseling, 25

D

daily life activities, 80
daily activities exercise, 76
day-to-day coping with PD,
    82–108
deep-brain stimulation
    (DBS) 64-67
    complications, 66
    good candidates, 66–67
    side effects, 66

deep breathing exercises,
    27
dementia with Lewy body
    disease, 15
denial, 16, 17
Deprenyl, 56
depression, 7, 22–25, 48, 55
    symptoms, 22, 23
diabetes, 52
diagnosing Parkinson's
    disease, 15–17
diarrhea, 55, 60
diet, 84–87
dietician, 50
dietitian, 39
digestive problems, 52
dizziness, 10, 51, 54, 57, 59,
    60, 102, 103
doctor prescribed activities,
    76
dopamine, 4, 6, 13, 48, 56,
    58
dopamine agonists, 52, 53
    side effects, 53
dressing and grooming,
    106, 107
driving, 35, 97
drooling, 48, 54, 60
drowsiness, 53, 54, 59
drug-allergy reactions, 61
drug reactions, 14, 47, 61
drug therapy, 47–63
drug tolerance, 47
drug treatment options,
    47–63
    benefits, 47
    side effects, 47
drugs for life, 63
durable power of attorney,
    119, 120
dyskinesia, 51, 55, 58
dystonia, 7, 58

E

Eldepryl, 56
electrical stimulation, 80
electrode, 66
electrode breakage, 66
Emory University School of
    Medicine, 71
emotional challenges,
    109–112
emotional side of
    Parkinson's disease,
    16–36
emotional support, 82–84
endogenous depression, 23
endorphins, 24, 72
enlarged pupils, 60
entacapone, 49, 58
environmental toxins, 14
enzyme inhibitors, 56–60
    types, 56
enzymes, 49, 56–60
excess salivation, 48
Exelon, 60
exercise, 71–82
    benefits, 72
    types, 76
exercise classes, 72
extremities weakness, 10

F

facial expression changes, 9
    see also hypomimia
fainting, 54, 102, 103
falling, 5
    prevention, 104, 105
fatigue, 23, 60
fever, 59
financial help, 118–119
food and drug interactions,
    50
free radicals, 14, 58

freezing, 67
freezing episodes, 8, 51

G

gait training, 80
genetic factors, 15
globus pallidus (GPi),
    65–67
guided imagery, 28

H

hallucinations, 54, 55, 57,
    60
handwriting changes, 9, 10
health care team, 38–40
    communication with, 43,
    44
heat and ice therapy, 80
HMO (health maintenance
    organization), 41
Huntington's disease, 15
hydrotherapy, 80
hyperactivity, 59
hypersexuality, 53, 98
hypokinetic dysarthria, 91
hypomimia, 48

I

inability to move, 8
incontinence, 101, 102
increased heart rate, 54
infection, 66
injection site discomfort, 53
insomnia, 23, 57
involuntary jerking, 51, 55
involuntary nodding, 51
irritability, 54, 55
isolation, 25, 72

J

jerky movements, 5, 51, 55
joint injury prevention, 72

K

Kemadrin, 54

L

l-dopa
  see levodpa
levodopa (l-dopa), 16, 17,
  48–52, 55–58
  combination with other
    drugs, 48, 49
  food and drug
    interactions, 50
  side effects, 48, 50–52
lightheadedness, 51, 59
liver function testing, 59
liver problems, 58
living will, 119
long-term care, 120–122
loss of appitite, 59
loss of energy, 23
loss of sex drive, 53
Lou Gehrig's disease, 13
low blood pressure, 102
low dopamine levels, 4
low-protein diets, 50

M

magnetic resonance
  imaging (MRI), 16, 64, 67
MAO-B inhibitors,
  monoamine oxidase type
  B (MAO-B) inhibitors,
  56, 57
marital and family
  counseling, 39
mask-like facial expressions
  see hypomimia

massage therapist, 39
Medic-Alert bracelet, 61
medication chart, 61
medication management,
  61, 62
medication safety, 61–63
meditation, 28
memory loss, 7, 10, 48, 54,
  55
mental disturbances, 38
mental health professional,
  17
microelectric recording, 64
Mirapex, 52
mood changes, 10, 55, 59
motor function, 5
motor system, 4
movement disorder, 38, 67
Movement Disorder Society
  (MDS), 57
MPTP, 14
multiple sclerosis, 13
multisystem atrophy, 15
muscle cramps, 51, 59
muscle injury prevention,
  72
muscle pain, 51, 59
muscle spasms, 7, 51, 59
muscle stiffness, 48
muscular dystrophy, 13

N

National Parkinson
  Foundation, 82, 83
nausea, 51, 55, 57, 59, 60
nerve cell damage, 13
nervous-system disorder, 38
neural implants, 70
neurologist, 38, 41
neurons, 4, 13, 56
neurostimulator, 66

neurosurgery, 64
neurotranmitters, 4
nightmares, 53, 55
nighttime leg cramping, 52
normal pressure
  hydrocephalis, 15

O

occupational therapies, 81
occupational therapist, 39
oily or dry skin, 9
"on-off" episodes, 50–52, 58
orthostatic hypotension, 57,
  102
outdated drugs, 63
oversleeping, 23
oxidants, 14

P

pain, 7, 10
pallidotomy, 67–69
  complications, 68
  good candidates, 68
Parkinson's disease
  causes, 13–15
  coping, 82–108
  defined, 4–17
  diagnosing, 15–17
  drug treatment options,
    23, 47–63
  stages, 10–12
  surgery treatment
    options, 64–70
  symptoms, 4–9, 43
Parkinson's Disease
  Foundation, 82
Parlodel, 52
partnership with doctors, 3,
  17, 37–46
passive exercises, 80
patient advocate, 44–46

PD-like symptoms, 15
PD research centers, 38, 41
PD support groups, 17, 24,
  40, 82–84
pesticide exposure, 14
pharmacist, 39, 40
physical challenges,
  114–116
physical therapist, 39
physical therapy, 80
pill cutter, 63
poor posture, 7
posture changes, 5, 10
pramipexole, 52
presymptomatic stage, 10
preventive exercises, 76
primary care physician, 38,
  41
procyclidine, 54
progressive supernuclear
  palsy, 15
protein in diet, 50
psychiatrist, 38, 39
psychotherapy, 39

Q

quality of life, 1, 75

R

rasagiline, 56, 57
realistic expectations, 75, 76
recreational exercises, 76
referrals, 40
Requip, 52
Requip XL, 52
resperine, 15
restless leg syndrome (RLS),
  103
restlessness, 23
rigidity, 7, 52, 64
rivastigmine, 60

side effects, 60
ropinirole, 52

S

safety at home, 104
sample exercise routine,
76–80
second opinions, 37
seizures, 60
selegiline, 56
selegiline hydrochloride, 56
self-help
elements, 1, 2
self-help approach, 1–3
sense of smell changes, 8,
10
serotonin, 23
sexual side effects, 53
sexuality issues, 97–102
side effects
amantadine, 55
anticholinergics, 54, 55
COMT inhibitors,
catechol-O-methyl-
transferase (COMT)
inhibitors, 59, 60
deep-brain stimulation,
66
dopamine agonists, 53
levodopa (l-dopa), 52
of medications, 43, 47
rivastigmine, 60
sexual, 53
tolcapone, 58, 59
signs of shock, 60
Sinemet, 48, 49, 58
Sinemet CR, 48
skin changes, 48, 55
sleeping difficulties, 9, 48,
55, 60, 87–91
slow movements, 52

slow thinking, 7
slowness of movement, 5
social worker, 39
sore throat, 59
speech changes, 8, 10
speech difficulties, 91–96
speech exercises, 93, 94
speech therapist, 39, 92
spiritual crisis, 113, 114
stages of Parkinson's
disease, 10–12
staging drugs, 47
Stalevo, 49, 58
stereotactic frame, 67
stiffness, 5, 10, 67
stomach problems, 52, 60
stooped posture, 5
strengthening exercising, 73
stress reduction, 25, 26
stretching exercise, 71, 73
substantia nigra, 6
subthalamic nucleus (STN),
65–66
suicidal thoughts, 23, 55
support groups, 17,
for caregivers, 109–122
surgery treatment options,
64–70
swallowing problems, 8,
91–96
signs, 95, 96
sweating, 53, 54, 60
Symmetrel, 55
symptoms of Parkinson's
disease, 4–9, 43

T

talking with your children,
32, 33
talking with your partner,
30–32

Tasmar, 58
telling your employer, 33,
	34
thalamotomy, 69–70
	complications, 69
	good candidates, 69–70
thalamus (Vim), 65–66, 69
tolcapone, 58
	side effects, 58, 59
tranquilizers, 15
traveling issues, 108
trembling, 51
tremor, 5, 48, 52, 64, 67
	drug to reduce, 53–55
trihexphenidyl HCI, 54
twitching, 51, 60
tyramine, 57

U

urinary problems, 8, 60

V

vision changes, 52, 96, 97

visual flashes, 66
vomiting, 60

W

walking impairment, 48
wearing-off effect, 50–52,
	58
weight loss, 23
Wilson's disease, 15
writing problems, 48

Y

yellowing of eyes or skin,
	59
yoga, 28, 75

Z

Zydis selegiline, 56

About the Authors

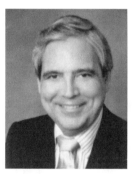

David **Cram, M.D.,** was diagnosed with Parkinson's disease in 1991. Consequently, he retired early from his practice as a dermatologist. Since his retirement, he has written four books. In addition to co-authoring the second edition of *Understanding Parkinson's Disease,* Dr. Cram is author of *Frequently Asked Questions about Parkinson's Disease* (Acorn Publishing, 2001), *Coping with Psoriasis* (Addicus Books, 2000), and *The Healing Touch—Keeping the Doctor-Patient Relationship Alive Under Managed Care* (Addicus Books, 1997).

Dr. Cram received his medical degree from the University of Wisconsin Medical School, Madison, Wisconsin, and trained for his dermatology specialty at the Mayo Clinic, Rochester, Minnesota. There, he earned a master of science in dermatology.

Upon completion of his medical training, he was assigned to the United States Air Force Base Hospital in Lakenheath, England, where he became chief of the Department of Medicine. During that time, he received the

Air Force Commendation Medal and rose to the rank of Lt. Colonel.

In 1971, Dr. Cram joined the staff of the University of California, San Francisco, where he became chief of the Dermatology Clinic, and served as a teacher, lecturer, and research scientist. After fifteen years in academia, Dr. Cram began a private practice in dermatology, which he maintained until 1991, when he was diagnosed with Parkinson's disease.

Dr. Cram is the author of dozens of scientific publications. Among his numerous honors and awards, he is credited with starting the first Psoriasis Day Care Treatment Center in the nation and was appointed clinical professor emeritus by the University of California in 1991.

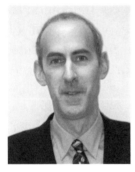

Steven H. Schechter, M.D., conducts his private practice as a neurologist in West Bloomfield, Michigan. He is board-certified by the American Board of Psychiatry and Neurology and by the American Board of Clinical Neurophysiology. Dr. Schechter is also a clinical assistant professor of neurology at Wayne State University.

A 1987 graduate of the Chicago Medical School at Rosalind Franklin University of Medicine and Science, he completed residencies in neurology at Henry Ford Hospital and Wayne State University School of Medicine and a postdoctoral fellowship in neurophysiology at the University of Michigan. He has been in practice since 1987 and has been affiliated with William Beaumont Hospital, Royal Oak, Michigan, in neurology since 1992.

Dr. Schechter's personal interests include bicycling, cooking, and gardening.

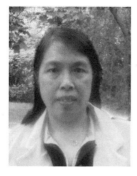

Xiao-Ke Gao, M.D., Ph.D., is a native of Beijing, China, where she earned her medical degree at Shanxi Medical College. She then went on to complete a master's degree in neuropsychopharmacology at the Beijing Academy of Medical Science. Dr. Gao earned her Ph.D. in neuropsychopharmacology at New York University (NYU) Medical Center's Department of Psychiatry. She remained in New York City, where she completed her neurology residency at NYU Medical Center. She then went on to pursue an EMG fellowship at Bellevue Hospital.

Following completion of residency training in neurology, Dr. Gao developed a practice in neurology in New York City with an emphasis on Parkinson's disease diagnostics and treatment. Motivated by her extensive patient experience and her own mother's condition of thirty years with Parkinson's disease, Dr. Gao has engineered dynamic pharmacology strategies suited to the individual Parkinson's patient. These optimize treatment response and minimize side effects and "tolerance" development. These strategies employ pharmacodynamic data-based adjustment of dosing over time, and at times can involve very low doses of two medications that act together to provide better benefit while minimizing side effects from either. Dr. Gao has developed quantitative methods to measure Parkinson's disease baseline symptom severity and treatment effects.

Dr. Gao has managed a successful private practice for more than eleven years and has expanded to two primary care clinics in midtown and Chinatown. In addition to her clinic work, Dr. Gao is an assistant professor of clinical neurology at NYU Medical Center. She currently acts as an attending physician at NYU Downtown Hospital, NYU Tisch Hospital, Bellevue Hospital, and St. Vincent's Hospital.

Dr. Gao can be reached through her Web site: www.easternneurologic.com.

Consumer Health Titles from Addicus Books
Visit our online catalog at www.AddicusBooks.com

After Mastectomy—Healing Physically and Emotionally . . . $14.95

Bariatric Plastic Surgery. $24.95

Body Contouring after Weight Loss $24.95

Cancers of the Mouth and Throat—
A Patient's Guide to Treatment. $14.95

Cataracts—A Patient's Guide to Treatment. $14.95

Cataract Surgery $19.95

Colon & Rectal Cancer—A Patient's Guide to Treatment . . . $14.95

Coping with Psoriasis—A Patient's Guide to Treatment. . . . $14.95

Coronary Heart Disease—
A Guide to Diagnosis and Treatment $15.95

Countdown to Baby $19.95

The Courtin Concept—Six Keys to Great Skin at Any Age . . $19.95

Elder Care Made Easier. $16.95

Exercising through Your Pregnancy. $19.95

Facial Feminization Surgery. $49.95

The Fertility Handbook—A Guide to Getting Pregnant $14.95

The Healing Touch—Keeping the Doctor/
Patient Relationship Alive under Managed Care $9.95

LASIK—A Guide to Laser Vision Correction $19.95

Living with P.C.O.S.—Polycystic Ovarian Syndrome $19.95

Look Out Cancer Here I Come $19.95

Lung Cancer—A Guide to Treatment & Diagnosis $14.95

The Macular Degeneration Source Book. $14.95

The New Fibromyalgia Remedy. $19.95

The Non-Surgical Facelift Book—
A Guide to Facial Rejuvenation Procedures $19.95

Overcoming Metabolic Syndrome $19.95

Overcoming Postpartum Depression and Anxiety $14.95

Overcoming Prescription Drug Addiction $19.95

Overcoming Urinary Incontinence. $19.95

A Patient's Guide to Dental Implants $14.95

Prostate Cancer—A Patient's Guide to Treatment $14.95

Sex and the Heart $19.95

Simple Changes—The Boomer's Guide
to a Healthier, Happier Life $9.95

A Simple Guide to Thyroid Disorders $14.95
Straight Talk about Breast Cancer—
  From Diagnosis to Recovery $15.95
The Stroke Recovery Book—
  A Guide for Patients and Families $14.95
The Surgery Handbook—
  A Guide to Understanding Your Operation $14.95
Understanding Lumpectomy—
  A Treatment Guide for Breast Cancer. $14.95
Understanding Parkinson's Disease—A Self-Help Guide . . . $19.95
Understanding Peyronie's Disease. $16.95
Understanding Your Living Will. $12.95
Your Complete Guide to Breast
  Augmentation & Body Contouring $21.95
Your Complete Guide to Breast Reduction & Breast Lifts . . $21.95
Your Complete Guide to Facial Cosmetic Surgery $19.95
Your Complete Guide to Facelifts. $21.95
Your Complete Guide to Nose Reshaping $21.95

To Order Books:

Visit us online at: www.addicusbooks.com
Call toll free: 800-352-2873

For discounts on bulk purchases, call our Special Sales Dept. at (402) 330-7493